Fats Are Good for You
and Other Secrets

Fats Are Good for You

AND OTHER SECRETS

HOW SATURATED FAT AND CHOLESTEROL
ACTUALLY BENEFIT THE BODY

Jon J. Kabara, PhD

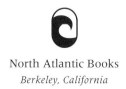

North Atlantic Books
Berkeley, California

Published by
North Atlantic Books   Cover photo © istockphoto.com
P.O. Box 12327   Cover and book design by Brad Greene
Berkeley, California 94712

Printed in the United States of America

Lauricidin® is a registered trademark of Jon J. Kabara.

Fats are Good for You and Other Secrets: How Saturated Fat and Cholesterol Actually Benefit the Body is sponsored by the Society for the Study of Native Arts and Sciences, a nonprofit educational corporation whose goals are to develop an educational and cross-cultural perspective linking various scientific, social, and artistic fields; to nurture a holistic view of arts, sciences, humanities, and healing; and to publish and distribute literature on the relationship of mind, body, and nature.

North Atlantic Books' publications are available through most bookstores. For further information, call 800-733-3000 or visit our website at www.northatlanticbooks.com.

Library of Congress Cataloging-in-Publication Data

Kabara, Jon J., 1926-
    Fats are good for you and other secrets : how saturated fat and cholesterol actually benefit the body / Jon J. Kabara.
        p. cm.
    Includes bibliographical references and index. Summary: "Presents infor-mation regarding the various roles played by fats and cholesterol in the body"—Provided by publisher.
    1. Saturated fatty acids in human nutrition—Popular works. 2. Choles-terol—Popular works. I. Title.
    ISBN 978-1-55643-690-1
    QP752.S37K33
    2007612'.01577—dc22
                                                          2007042453
                                                          CIP

1 2 3 4 5 6 7 8 9 VERSA 14 13 12 11 10 09 08

Table of Contents

Acknowledgments

I'm grateful to my many colleagues who over the years supported and encouraged my research efforts. To name but a few:

Jeffrey Andrews

Conrado Dayrit, MD

Hans Kaunitz, MD

Lon Lewis, DVM

Donald Orth, PhD

Jacquelyn McCandless, MD

Rachael Schemmel, PhD

Charles Tweedle, PhD

John Upledger, DO

Van D. Merkle, DC

Vermen M. Verallo-Rowell, MD

Andrew Weil, MD

In addition, I wish to give credit to all my students who in reality taught me more than I taught them. My family made many sacrifices so that I could obtain my degrees (BS, MS, and PhD) and spend research time away from them. They should take credit and solace for all that has been accomplished through the research on cholesterol and the saturated lipid monolaurin, sold as an approved food supplement called Lauricidin. Without the continued love and support from Betty, my wife, and the efforts of my grandson Brian Kabara, the Lauricidin story would never have been written.

—Jon J. Kabara, 2007

Preface

This book represents the culmination of my fifty-plus years of research on lipids. I primarily studied cholesterol, one of several lipid types in the human body. Put simply, "lipid" is a generic term encompassing compounds that are mostly water-insoluble. Lipids found in the human body include a variety of substances like fatty acids, phospholipids, triglycerides (fats), and cholesterol. Fats may be solid at room temperature or liquid; in the latter case they are called "oils."

This book is part of an ongoing story, with much still to learn, including better ways to nourish and heal our bodies. It is my hope that this book will stimulate more research on the topics, since our knowledge of saturated fats and cholesterol and their health benefits is far from complete.

The question of whether or not fats are "good" or "bad" for us has occupied me since I was a graduate student. While attending the University of Chicago, my doctoral thesis topic was the relationship between cholesterol and cancer. As a doctoral student I was privileged to work under the tutelage of George V. Leroy, MD, and to be part of the first (1955) studies on the metabolism of cholesterol in humans using radioactive C14-H3 labeled acetate. One of my teachers was Conrad Block, PhD, who received the Nobel Prize for his work on how the body makes cholesterol. Another aspect of fats/lipids involves other lipids (besides cholesterol) like fatty acids and monoglycerides, and their antimicrobial properties.

From these early experiences, it was evident to me that cholesterol and certain saturated fats are necessary for optimal health. It has been frustrating to read constantly (for fifty years) that cholesterol and saturated fats were considered to be major contributors to various health problems. From my extensive studies involving cholesterol, I found it hard to believe that cholesterol is the culprit that so many health professionals make it out to be. In the evolution of animal life, cholesterol formation occurred only when oxygen was first available. A teleology argument would suggest that Nature would not allow cholesterol to be formed unless it had a useful purpose. In fact, it has now been shown that cholesterol is not only found in high concentrations in the brain and nerve tissue, it also is the precursor of bile acids involved in fat digestion. Other derivatives of cholesterol are male and female sex hormones, steroid hormones, and vitamin D. In addition, cholesterol is essential for the formation of all cell membranes and helps maintain their integrity.

Fats have been mostly discussed from the point of view of calories alone, in both the scientific literature and popular writing. To emphasize a greater role for lipids and fats, I edited three volumes on the pharmacological roles of these two nutrients, published in 1978, 1985, and 1989 by the American Oil Chemists' Society. (These volumes are referenced in a few places throughout the present book; see also Bibliography A.)

Contrary to popular notions found in both lay and medical press, cholesterol is not a villain to human health. Cholesterol is not only found in all cells of the body, it is the precursor to a variety of hormones like adrenal steroids, the male testosterone, and the female estrogen. In addition, as will be explained later in the book, cholesterol actually acts as part of a protective mechanism against blood vessel injury.

In addition to refuting the claimed danger of cholesterol, the other important message of this book is that *not all saturated fats are the same or even "bad."* The term "saturated fat" is ambiguous since it includes a family of three (short-, medium-, and long-carbon chain) saturated fatty acids, all of which have different properties. Certain medium-chain saturated fats (coconut oil and palm kernel oil, for example) can't be all bad since almost half the world's population—represented by China, India, and the Pacific Rim islands—consumes these fats in the form of tropical oils. Coconut oil in a *balanced* diet of fish, vegetables, and fruit, etc., is healthy saturated oil.

While various aspects of lipid/fat chemistry and biochemistry will be related to diseases, the main "player" in this story is a saturated lipid called monolaurin; the registered brand name for high-quality monolaurin produced in a laboratory I established is Lauricidin. The exact chemical names for Lauricidin are glyceryl monolaurate, sn-1 monolaurin, or simply monolaurin. Since commercial monolaurins are normally only 50% pure, I chose the name Lauricidin and trademarked this substance to emphasize the crucial importance of the high purity of the monolaurin that our group and others used in their lipid/fat research. In this book, the two names monolaurin and Lauricidin are used to refer to the same thing, despite the fact that commercial versions are not equivalent.

As I researched the antimicrobial and other properties of lipids, it became evident that monoglycerides are important products found in nature. Some natural sources for saturated monoglycerides are mother's milk, saw palmetto, bitter melon, and a minor component of virgin coconut oil.

The *nutriceutical* (nutritional and healing properties of a food additive) effects of monolaurin include antibacterial, antifungal/antiyeast, and antiviral. These properties offer a unique alternative to drugs, especially antibiotics. The effects of monolaurin, a saturated fat, include extraordinary health benefits without the danger of toxicity, bacterial resistance formation, or negative interaction with most drugs or other supplements.

Monolaurin is a nutritional supplement for the whole family, including pets. The extraordinary numbers of unsolicited testimonials I have received speak loudly of the benefits it provides. While not hard-core scientific evidence, numerous testimonial letters supporting benefits in various health conditions using monolaurin cannot simply be disregarded as a "placebo effect."

Introduction to Fats/Oils

A common misconception often held by food writers, members of the general public, and even health professionals is that saturated fats and oils need to be avoided or reduced in our diet. This is not completely true. First, as mentioned above, there are three kinds of saturated fats: short-, medium-, and long-chain saturated fats. Each has different and important roles in promoting our good health. Second, all fats are healthy and necessary *if* combined in a balanced way.

Let's discuss the terms "fats" and "lipids" so we can be clear about our topic. Lipids, the catchall or generic label, are a family of substances (steroids, cholesterol, triglycerides, phospholipids, etc.) not soluble in water. The term "fat," although the substance is considered a lipid, is restricted to a compound that has three fatty acids attached to a glycerol molecule; the resulting chemical is called a triglyceride. A solid triglyceride is called a "fat," while a triglyceride that melts at room temperature is called "oil."

For visualization, a triglyceride is composed of glycerol and three fatty acids joined as in the structural diagram below.

```
 H                                              H
H-C-OH sn1  position                           H-C-OR
H-C-OH sn2  position  +  3 CH3-(CH2)n-COOH  =  H-C-OR
H-C-OH sn3  position                           H-C-OR
 H                                              H
Glycerol              +  3 Fatty acids(OR)  =  Triglyceride
```

In this illustration, *sn* represents the glycerol carbon position; *n* and *R* the length and kind of fatty acid attached to glycerol. If the majority of the fatty acids are saturated, then the triglyceride is a solid fat. If the majority are not unsaturated, then the triglyceride is an oil. Where there are two fatty acids attached to glycerol, the lipid is now known as a *diglyceride* (DG). A *monoglyceride* (MG) lipid—of which there are two kinds—will have only one fatty acid attached to the sn1(3) or the sn2 position of glycerol. The fatty acids in the sn1 and sn3 positions are similar since they occupy a position at either end of the glycerol molecule. Therefore, not all monoglycerides are the same since the fatty acid can occupy the end position—sn1(3)—of glycerol or the middle sn2 position. Later their structural differences will be emphasized. It is important therefore to remember these structural sn designations since they reflect the different biological metabolism of the two monoglycerides.

In lipid biochemistry, all fatty acids are classified according to the number of carbon atoms present in their structure, as well as the degree of saturation, which refers to how many hydrogen atoms are bonded to the carbons.

Saturated fatty acids are chains of carbon and hydrogen atoms strung together like a beaded necklace with an acid, chemically known as a carboxyl group (COOH), attached to one end of the carbon chain. Each carbon atom needs two hydrogen atoms, except the end carbon, which has three hydrogen atoms.

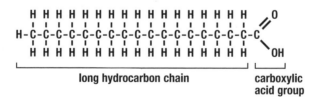

long hydrocarbon chain   carboxylic acid group

A fat like oleic acid with two hydrogens missing is *monounsaturated.*

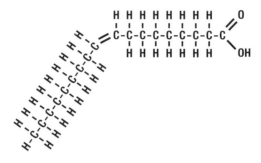

A fat such as linoleic with two double bonds has four hydrogens missing and is called a *polyunsaturated* fatty acid.

Long-chain (more than 14 carbon atoms, represented as >C14) saturated fatty acids predominate principally in animal fats, while palm kernel and coconut oils are noted to contain predominantly medium-chain (C8-C12) saturated fatty acids. Monounsaturated fatty acids abound in nuts, avocados, olive oil, and surprisingly in some animal fats (especially pig fat or lard).

Polyunsaturated fatty acids are mostly found in vegetable oils, but significant amounts are found in fish oils and chicken skin. The human body needs but cannot synthesize some polyunsaturated fats. These necessary dietary fats are called essential fatty acids (EFAs).

All fats and oils, whether of animal or vegetable origin, tend to be blends of these three types of fatty acids, with one fatty acid usually predominating, depending on the food.

It should be noted here that saturated fats are the most chemically stable fat. Even monounsaturated fats do not go rancid (i.e., oxidize) easily if stored properly. Likewise, these fats are more stable under heat, making them ideal for cooking. Polyunsaturated fats, however, especially those of vegetable origin, are not as stable and go rancid more quickly, even in the body. Rancid oils breed cancer-causing and tissue-damaging free radicals. Thus, polyunsaturated fats should not exceed about 15% of our total caloric intake due to the propensity for free radical formation.

The two essential fatty acids that we obtain from polyunsaturated fats are linolenic (an omega-3 fatty acid) and linoleic (an omega-6 fatty acid). The "3" and "6" indicate where the first double bond occurs in the fatty acid chain.

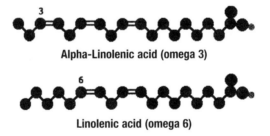

Alpha-Linolenic acid (omega 3)

Linolenic acid (omega 6)

The body takes omega-3 and -6 fatty acids and creates hormone-like substances called prostaglandins that can carry out a host of metabolic functions. Like vitamins and minerals, EFAs must be obtained from our food. In times past, humans consumed a balance of linolenic and other omega-3 fatty acids (found principally in cold-water fish, walnuts, eggs, flax oil, dark-green leafy vegetables, cod liver oil, and some whole grains) as well as linoleic and other omega-6 fatty acids (found principally in vegetables). This is as it should be, since both are critically important. An overabundance of one kind of fat, as you will learn reading this book, can cause a host of undesirable reactions including sexual and immune dysfunction, as well as increased cancer risk. So while the quality and variety of fats are more important than the quantity (something dieters need to realize), this is not an endorsement to overeat fat!

This book explains the beneficial effects on our health and healing that occur via consumption of sn1-monoglycerides and/or sn3-monoglycerides (commonly shortened to sn1(3)-monoglycerides) of saturated medium-chain length (C8, C10, and particularly C12 monoglyceride, a.k.a. Lauricidin). As mentioned, these fats are found in mother's milk, saw palmetto, bitter melon, and as a minor component in virgin coconut oil. The recommended dietary supplement is Lauricidin, which can be obtained from your health professional or by going to www.Lauricidin.com.

In 2004 authors from the Department of Food Science and Technology at the University of California wrote: "The evidence is not strong that overall dietary intervention by lowering saturated fat intake lowers the incidence of nonfatal coronary artery disease (CAD), total mortality, or prolongs life." (German and Dillard 2004)

Countless studies show that the *more* animal fats people eat, the better their heart health. Proof from the real world? The African Masai, North American Eskimos, Japanese, Greeks, and French consume diets that are extremely high in saturated animal fats. Yet these groups enjoy astonishingly low rates of heart disease, hypertension, and coronary events.

The above is *not* an endorsement to eat as much fat as possible. Good nutrition, always a balance of different food groups, depends on not only the foods we eat but also our individual genetic makeup. "One diet size does not fit all."

What the above does recommend, however, is a putting aside of past theories of the ill effects of saturated lipids. Allow these new facts about saturated fats and cholesterol to be integrated with your awareness of your dietary experience. You may conclude, as I have, that it is "time for an oil change," both in our thinking and in our diet.

Thomas H. Huxley (1825–1895) observed "the great tragedy of science—the slaying of a beautiful theory by an ugly fact."

This observation can certainly be applied to the theoretical view that saturated fats and cholesterol are bad for our health. Perhaps my pointing out "ugly facts" will disprove this theory finally.

Nature provides us with a variety of substances that result in better health and self-healing. Fats in general—and certain saturated fats in particular—help our bodies to a state of wellness. Wellness is more than the absence of disease. It is the state of being in our best possible physical and mental condition.

The abundance of documented scientific facts reviewed in this book will tell, as radio personality Paul Harvey would say, "the rest of the story." The truth is that saturated fats and cholesterol are not all bad. It needs to be repeated that the term "saturated" refers not to a single entity but rather a group of three families of fats. Saturated fats are chemically classified into three primary categories based on their carbon chain length: short (C2-C6), medium (C8-C12), or long (C14 or greater). Each sub-group has markedly different caloric and pharmacological effects that are not recognized, even in most science and medical journals. The term "saturated" when used should always be prefixed by an adjective (short-, medium-, or long-chain).

Currently there is renewed interest in examining natural substances for ingredients or properties that can keep us healthy and aid the body in healing more rapidly. Drugs, which are useful, are not always an answer for keeping disease at bay. Most drugs affect symptoms and not causes. As will be discussed later, lipid-lowering drugs like statins are a good example of undesirable drug side effects. The consequences of taking drugs may present more danger than high cholesterol levels. The highly respected *Journal of the American Medical Association* (Volume 279, April 1998) stated that prescription medications kill close to 200,000 people a year, making adverse drug reactions the fourth leading cause of death in the United States. The Seventh Annual Conference on Anti-Aging Medicine announced that according to a survey done by the *New England Journal of Medicine,* 77% of Americans would prefer natural treatments rather than prescription drugs.

Overall, 51% of *approved* drugs have serious side effects not detected prior to drug approval. Not only is that astounding, but 59% of the people surveyed said they would change doctors if they could find one who would utilize natural therapies before resorting to prescription drugs. Does that tell you something about the problems of current treatments with drugs? On the other hand, many natural medicines by competent herbalists have been used for centuries without negative side effects.

It is important to emphasize that fats/lipids can influence our hormonal status and modify cell membrane structure and function, as well as cell-signaling transduction pathways and gene expression. Simple lipids can influence the function of the immune system. Fats/lipids need to be considered for more than their calorie content. The effect of a fat (or any nutrient) depends on our genetic requirements (nutrigenomics). One's individual requirement for a nutrient can vary greatly among different people.

CHAPTER 1

Historical Notes on Natural Medicines

Nature, which provides a cornucopia of healing substances, is the basis of both traditional Chinese medicine and Ayurveda (an ancient Hindu treatise on the art of healing and prolonging life). It was as a young student of pharmacology at the University of Chicago that I was first impressed by the fact that almost every modern drug is based on findings in nature. In contrast to Western medicinal chemicals, the benefits of natural products are not always subjected to the golden rule of "controlled clinical/double blind studies." Thus, their efficacy is often considered anecdotal, not absolute. Modern medicines developed in the laboratory are usually made up of single components, very concentrated, and designed to work quickly. The results are sometimes dramatic. However, the very real risks of negative side effects with these drugs are greater than with natural supplements.

In the last couple of decades, there has been an increased interest (again) in natural products on the part of the scientific establishment, with renewed credence given to their potential. These products from natural sources are seen as a means of identifying new and novel pharmacological compounds that could be useful in clinical medicine. It has long been known that nature offers substances that can attack disease and improve our health, often at a reduced cost and with fewer side effects than a pharmaceutical approach.

I can imagine the treatment dilemma of an ancient medicine man or woman who, without the benefit of controlled studies for natural substances, was guided only by vague symptoms such as a generalized pain, nausea, fever, or convulsions. In such a predicament, and with little if any scientific knowledge of anatomy or pathology, early healers administered herbal concoctions in the hope that they would work. The medicine man undoubtedly added prayers or exorcisms to the medication and believed sincerely that his ministrations would aid the afflicted. Fortunately, some medicine men and women were careful observers, with a patient's recovery uppermost in mind. Successful healers with a scientific bent and/or deep compassion were likely to have searched for valid explanations of their findings.

Today we need to return to similar validation studies, since funding for "controlled studies" like those carried out for new drugs is usually not available for food supplements like Lauricidin. Current federal government studies focused on testing natural substances as alternative medicines are primarily designed to find fault with the natural supplement as opposed to support for its continued use. This negative attitude is fostered by the pharmaceutical industry with obvious economic motives: natural supplements like Lauricidin cannot be easily patented or exploited, and their successful use threatens the profits of drug-makers.

One of the oldest records of useful natural medicines is found in the writings of the Chinese scholar-emperor Shen Nung, who lived almost five thousand years ago (2735 BC). He compiled a book on natural substances called *The Yellow Emperor's Classic of Internal Medicine,* a forerunner of the medieval pharmacopoeia that listed all the then-known medications. One of the more important substances listed in the Chinese classic was bufotoxin, found in the glands of toads. Although toxic, bufotoxin has been used by the Chinese to treat heart problems. Bufotoxin, similar to digitalis, contains substances like epinephrine (adrenaline) and norepinephrine. Digitalis, the drug, is currently used to strengthen heart muscle to avoid congestive heart failure.

Other examples of gifts from nature are two South American plants containing substances known as alkaloids. They have gained worldwide importance as modern drugs. These extracts are cocaine and quinine.

Cocaine, the primary alkaloid, is extracted from leaves, especially from *Erythroxylum coca,* a bushy shrub native to South American countries at high altitudes, including Colombia, Bolivia, Peru, Ecuador, and Chile. Cocaine's potential for addiction was known and used with sinister intent by South American Indian chiefs hundreds of years ago. The chiefs maintained a messenger system along the spine of the Andes to control their thinly populated kingdoms. Their cities stretched for thousands of miles along the mountains and were isolated from each other by the rugged terrain. The messengers had to run at high altitudes and needed stimulants for this exhausting task. In payment for their feat, they were given more cocaine and thus were "owned by the company store" and their loyalty ensured.

Sigmund Freud, the Austrian psychoanalyst (1856–1939), treated many deeply disturbed cocaine addicts. In the course of his practice, he noted the numbing effect of the drug. He called this effect to the attention of the clinical pharmacologist Carl Koller, who introduced cocaine as a local anesthetic for surgical procedures.

The other important alkaloid was quinine. The Peruvian Indians had recognized for years the value of the quinquina tree for treating feverish patients (using the bark). A persistent story exists about Doña Francisca Henriquez de Ribera, wife of Count Chinchon, the Spanish viceroy of Peru. She fell ill with malaria (the "tertians" variety, with chills and fever that recur every third day). An Indian healer who gave her the bark cured her. In gratitude for the cure, the countess distributed the bark to other patients in Lima and thus alerted Spanish physicians to its clinical potential. The great Swedish botanist Carl Linnaeus (1707–1778) later called the tree "cinchona" in honor of Countess Chinchon, misspelling her name in the process. Two hundred years after the bark was introduced into Europe for the treatment of malaria, quinine (the actual chemical) was isolated from the bark of the cinchona tree by two French chemists, Caventou and Pelletier, in 1820.

While best known, the cinchona tree is not the only source of quinine. There is one tree family in North America that also contains traceable amounts of this alkaloid. The tree family Rubiaceae, a widely distributed family of mostly tropical trees, shrubs, and herbs, includes coffee, cinchona, and gardenia. The well-known magnolia tree that grows in swampy areas in the southeastern United States surprisingly contains quinine. By finding small amounts of quinine in these plant extracts, I recorded the first unpublished report to give credence to the magnolia's Indian name of "Fever Tree." The amount of quinine found, however, was less than 0.05% and of little commercial value.

One of the most important substances found in nature is salicin. The synthetic chemical compound derived from salicin is better known as aspirin. It is made from salicylic acid, found in the bark of the willow tree. Willow bark was mentioned in ancient texts from Assyria, Sumeria, and Egypt as a remedy for aches and fever, and the Greek physician Hippocrates wrote about its medicinal properties in the fifth century BC. Native Americans throughout the Western hemisphere relied on it as a staple of their medical treatments. The active extract of the bark, salicin, was isolated to its crystalline form in 1828 by Henri Leroux, a French pharmacist, and Raffaele Piria, an Italian chemist, who then succeeded in separating out the acid in its pure state. A saturated solution of salicin in water is acidic (pH = 2.4). Because of the low pH, salicin is called salicylic acid.

In 1897, German researcher Felix Hoffmann created a synthetically altered version of salicin (in his case, derived from the Spiraea plant), which caused less digestive upset than pure salicylic acid. The new drug, formally labeled acetylsalicylic acid, was named "aspirin" by Hoffmann's employer, Bayer AG. This gave rise to the hugely important class of drugs known as non-steroidal anti-inflammatory drugs (NSAIDs).

The notion that "natural" products are not toxic is simplistic and naïve. Two natural products that come to mind are cobra venom, which I worked with while at the University of Miami (*Cobras In My Garden,* by Bill Haas), and digitalis. The latter is a cardioactive or cardiotonic steroid-like drug that has the ability to exert a specific and powerful strengthening of cardiac muscle.

Digitalis was first used to treat "dropsy," once a widespread illness in which water filtered into every available space and expanded the body like a balloon into grotesque shapes. Sometimes the liquid—quarts and gallons of it—made arms and legs swell so that they were immovable. The modern "discovery" of digitalis is credited to the Scottish doctor William Withering. While working as a physician in Staffordshire in the eighteenth century, his girlfriend got him so interested in plants and botany that in 1776 he published a huge treatise, the title of which is *A Botanical Arrangement of All the Vegetables Growing in Great Britain.* But prior to the book's publication, one of Withering's patients came to him in 1775 with a very bad heart condition, and since Withering had no effective treatment for him, he told the patient that he was going to die. The patient, being an independent type, went to a local gypsy, took a secret herbal remedy, and promptly got much better!

When Withering heard about this, he became quite excited and searched for the gypsy throughout the byways of Shropshire. Eventually he found her and demanded to know what was in the secret remedy. After much bargaining, the gypsy finally told her secret. The herbal remedy was made from a whole concoction of things, but the active ingredient was the purple foxglove, *Digitalis purpurea.* The potency of digitalis extract had been known since the Dark Ages, when it was used as a poison for the medieval "trial by ordeal," and also used as an external application to promote the healing of wounds.

William Withering gave a succinct description of digitalis toxicity. The glycoside component of the substance (a chemical compound that when cleaved breaks into a steroid portion much like cholesterol) continues to be the source of the most prevalent "iatrogenic" intoxication, a term used to describe a symptom or illness brought on unintentionally by something that a doctor does or says. Although the true incidence is currently unknown, studies in the 1960s and 1970s indicated that about 20% of hospitalized patients taking digitalis suffered definite digitalis toxicity, of which as many as 41% died. Today a better understanding of digitalis pharmacokinetics, drug interactions, smaller maintenance doses, and better utilization of serum levels has since reduced the occurrence of drug toxicity with digitalis.

Relative to our appreciation for healthful lipids/fats is mother's breast milk, another natural "product" that contains a host of valuable substances with nutritional and medical properties. Such products are now called "nutriceuticals" to refer to a food that has both nutritional value and pharmacological (medical) effects as well. Mother's milk could be called the first nutriceutical, since it not only provides important nutrients for growth and development of the infant, but also special medium-chain lipids/fats that have antimicrobial protective properties beneficial to the newborn.

This book highlights some of the nutriceutical properties found in mother's milk, saw palmetto, bitter melon, and a minor component of crude tropical oils. In older Asian civilizations, these foods were noted both for their nutritional and medical benefits. These diverse natural sources have nutriceutical effects that are similar because of their saturated monoglyceride content.

CHAPTER 2

Metabolism of Fats

This section aims to refute erroneous information found frequently on the Internet purporting that since a fat like coconut oil contains certain biologically active medium-chain fatty acids (like lauric acid), the beneficial ingredients are automatically available for medicinal purposes. These assertions are not true. This is like saying that since banks store money, the money is readily available to everyone. The fatty acid of the monoglyceride formed from a fat, which is a triglyceride, is found in the human body in the sn2 position; while the fatty acid in preformed (chemically synthesized) monoglyceride (Lauricidin) is in the sn1(3) position. These two monoglycerides are distinct and have different pharmacological actions, as will be explained.

Absorption and Digestion of Fats

For effective absorption into the body, dietary fats (triglycerides, or TG) need to be present in the intestines as sn2-monoglyceride, the absorbable form with two free fatty acids. Any absorbed monoglyceride is reformed by intestinal cells into a newly configured TG that is structurally different from the initial TG. The reformulated TG is then excreted into the lymphatic or portal blood system (which serves the liver) and transported throughout the body. In normal absorption, the mechanism and efficiency of each step depends on the fatty acid composition of the food.

Long-chain fatty acids (ingested as fats) are made soluble by micelle (particle, globular) formation and transported to the lymphatic system. In this respect, unsaturated fatty acids are more completely absorbed than long-chain saturated fats. In contrast, short- and medium-chain fatty acids are more soluble and absorbed as such by the intestinal cells. From these cells, they are removed via the portal system.

Fat digestion results in a mixture of sn2-monoglycerides and two fatty acids. The sn2-monoglyceride and the two free fatty acids are absorbed and then reassembled randomly into a new triglyceride (TG). Synthetic (laboratory-made) sn1-monoglycerides like monolaurin, however, are metabolized in a different way from the absorbed components of TG. *Monolaurin, the sn1(3)-monoglyceride, is not reesterified into an inactive TG.* It should be emphasized that after ingestion of high-quality monolaurin, fat particles (chylomicrons) are not observed in the blood as they are after ingestion of other fats. With fat ingestion, hyperglyceridemia or chylomicronemia occurs since the fats are reformed into new TGs in the blood. Reformation into TGs does not happen after intake of the sn1-monoglyceride as it does after the digestion of other fats.

The rise and duration of fat globules in the blood is greater after consumption of long-chain fats than after medium-chain fats. As stated above, the two fatty acids and sn2-monoglycerides formed during most fat digestion are absorbed in mucosal intestinal cells and resynthesized into new triglycerides. The fatty acid in the sn2 position of the monoglyceride, however, remains in place during this process. The reader needs to put the above explanation of lipid metabolism into perspective since the biological effects of any fatty acid in a fat depend on its position on the glycerol skeleton. Different fatty acids are absorbed at different rates and in varying amounts of the total. Therefore, nutritional statements concerning the amount of saturated fat in the diet are meaningless since they don't reflect how much is absorbed. Whether saturated fats contain short-chain fatty acids, medium-chain fatty acids, or long-chain fatty acids, and depending upon the position of the fatty acids on the glycerol backbone, saturated fats will have different physiological effects.

Metabolic Fate of Triglycerides (TGs)

Triglycerides are metabolized into two fatty acids and an sn2-monoglyceride by an enzyme catalyst called lipase. (TGs are formed then broken down then reformed again, but not by the same fatty acids.) This breakdown of the TG occurs in the mouth, stomach, and small intestine. These water-insoluble lipids are attached to proteins to form water-soluble lipoproteins. The products of hydrolysis are further packaged along with lipoprotein and other components into fat globules. These oil-in-water emulsions (a suspension of fats in water) are broken down by the lipase enzyme in the stomach. Gastric lipase preferentially hydrolyzes short- and medium-chain fatty acids from the sn3 position of the TG. As the lipid mixture passes into the small intestine, pancreatic lipase may then hydrolyze the sn1 and sn3 positions of the diglyceride. The products of this final reaction are two free fatty acids and an sn2-monoglyceride.

After absorption, the two free fatty acids and sn2-monoglyceride available are of special interest. Short- and medium-chain fatty acids and monoglycerides are absorbed into the portal vein and immediately transported to the liver. Long-chain (>C14) fatty acids are better absorbed if present in the sn2 position. This is particularly true when calcium is present, since the combination of calcium and free or unbound long-chain fatty acids results in a poorly soluble fatty acid salt. What we call "hard water," for example, is due to the presence of minerals that can form insoluble compounds with long-chain fatty acids.

In the typical scenario for the digestion and absorption of triglycerides (fats), the type of fatty acids released from the sn1 and sn3 positions often have different metabolic fates. Short- and medium-chain fatty acids can be solubilized in the water phase of the intestinal contents, where they are absorbed, bound to a protein like albumin, and transported directly to the liver via the portal vein. The location of long-chain fatty acids on the glycerol molecule of the TG can influence their metabolic destiny. When acids such as palmitic (C16) and stearic acid (C18) occupy the sn1 and sn3 terminal positions and are then removed from the TG, they have a low level of absorption because of their ability to form insoluble mineral salts. Therefore, fats that have long-chain saturated fatty acids in the sn1 and sn3 positions of triglycerides may exhibit different absorption/ dietary patterns than fats with palmitic or stearic acids in the middle sn2 position that are absorbed intact with the glycerol. It's a good example of the "old saw" theory that it's not what we ingest but what we absorb that is important. The effect of calcium forming an insoluble soap best illustrates this scenario.

The Effects of Fats on Calcium Absorption

Long-chain saturated fatty acids in the sn1(3) position of a TG form calcium soaps that are ten to twenty times less soluble than the calcium salts of unsaturated acids like oleic (C18:2) and linoleic (C18:3). Research has shown that high-calcium fortification (2,200 mg/day) in a diet that derives 34% of its energy from saturated fat (primarily beef tallow) decreases both saturated fat and calcium absorption. Calcium fortification decreased long-chain fatty acid absorption, total serum cholesterol, and LDL cholesterol compared with the low-calcium diet (Lukaski and Johnson, in Ching Kuang Chow, editor). Individuals taking calcium should take the supplement prior to and not after a heavy-fat meal. The calcium soaps that may form are not easily absorbed.

To reiterate my point, the position of a fatty acid on the glycerin structure influences absorption. Manufacturers of specialty foods designed to provide high-calorie intake (e.g. infant formulas and enteral supplements) should be aware of positional fatty acid distribution and utilize more fats that have short- or medium-chain saturated fatty acids at the sn1(3) location on the triglyceride. Conversely, food manufacturers should take advantage of the medium-chain triglyceride oils (often referred to as "MCT oils") to produce dietary products. These fats have approximately 10% less caloric value than long-chain fats and are not deposited in adipose tissue. In a balanced diet medium-chain triglycerides have less adverse effects on atherosclerosis markers such as blood triglycerides and cholesterol levels than do long-chain saturated fats.

CHAPTER 3

Lipids as Antimicrobial Agents

The objective of this chapter is to collate and evaluate the literature concerning antimicrobial lipids. Triglycerides (TGs) are either solid (fats) or liquid (oils) at room temperature. While TGs are not antimicrobially active, their free, non-esterified fatty acids have a long history of use as antimicrobial agents. Soaps (i.e., sodium or potassium salts of fatty acids) have been used as cleaning and disinfecting agents for centuries. Before 1930, the lack of success in the search for active antibacterial agents other than fatty acids resulted in pessimism as to whether an active antimicrobial agent would ever be found.

Two important discoveries, however, changed the course of thinking on the subject. The first was a serendipitous finding by British researcher Alexander Fleming, who in 1928 observed the lysis (breakdown) of Staphylococcus colonies in an area surrounding the growth of Penicillium, a mold. From this observation, new biochemical structures called antibiotics were added to the small arsenal of organic and inorganic compounds known to be lethal to microorganisms.

The second event was the discovery of a synthetic (lab-made) group of antimicrobials named sulfonamides. Trefouel, Nitti, and Boret in Fourneau's laboratory at the Pasteur Institute in France first observed these in 1935. This discovery enhanced hope for finding new and more effective synthetic antimicrobial agents; and in less than a decade, these two important discoveries together gave tremendous impetus to the search for new antimicrobial agents. The biocidal activity (killing power) of the newly isolated antibiotics and synthesized germicides was much greater than that of fatty acids. In proportion to the speed with which new and more powerful antibiotics and useful synthetic products were discovered, interest in the action of lipid germicides waned.

However, the use of these more powerful "magic bullets" is accompanied by complications. First, antibiotics and synthetic germicides are not without health risks in terms of toxicity, irritation, allergic reactions, and the possible development of bacterial resistance. Second, the long-term cost of these newer agents precludes their use in quantities normally required except in special situations. Third, the overuse (often in inappropriate-use circumstances) of these germicides has caused resistant organisms to appear. Because of these limitations, I became interested in safer and more effective antimicrobial agents that might be found in nature. Following is a brief history of the use of fatty acids as antimicrobials and our discovery of a high-quality monolaurin (Lauricidin), which is a safe and useful antimicrobial agent for better health.

Fatty Acids as Antimicrobial Agents

Some fatty acids found in nature have played an important historical role in food preservation. The old standbys (e.g. vinegar—about

4% acetic acid—from ancient Egypt) have been supplemented over the years by many fatty acids that are more active. These include sorbic acid, isolated from rowanberry oil and reported in 1859 by H. Hoffman; benzoic acid discovered by H. Fleck in 1875; and propionic acid, all useful in food preservation.

The organic acids described above are generally employed in products as acidulants (substances used to control pH), co-emulsifiers, or super-fatting agents. The latter property is used to replace the natural lipids of our skin. Stearic acid is the fatty acid most often used in the cosmetic industry. Because there are at least a hundred fatty acids available to the formulator, we are led to wonder what special benefit to product integrity and consumer needs could be satisfied by different fatty acids. The answer to this simple question was the basis of my own fifty-plus years of research relating the role of fatty acid structure to biological effects. While interest in the antimicrobial benefits of fatty acids in consumer products has been appreciated, I became aware that the antimicrobial activity of the fatty acid in human health should be reconsidered. My detailed studies of structure in relation to antimicrobial effects of lipid derivatives (fatty acids and their corresponding mono-esters) have been published in an American Oil Chemists' Society monograph *(The Pharmacological Effects of Lipids,* Vol. I, Ch. 1, pp. 1–14). The materials presented in this chapter attempt to summarize the contribution of fatty acid and ester structure to antimicrobial function.

Historically much of the early research on the germicidal activity of fatty acids was carried out between 1920 and 1940. I reviewed more up-to-date studies in this field (see Kabara 1978, 1984, and 1997 in the references list towards the back of the book).

One of the easiest ways to control the growth of microorganisms is by pH (a measure of acidity or alkalinity). Microorganisms have specific pH requirements for growth. As antimicrobial agents, fatty acids have their optimum antimicrobial action at low pH (high acid content). At neutral pH values (water has a neutral pH of 7.0) or higher (>pH 7.0), fatty acids are less effective antimicrobials. In addition, the structure of the fatty acid is all-important. This can be seen in Table 3.1.

One of the problems in earlier studies using fatty acids, however, was the dubious purity of the compounds being tested. For example, the unsaturated fatty acids were not tested for peroxide formation and seldom were chromatographically pure. Support for this statement comes from evaluating the potency of pure arachidonic acid. Kabara et al. found no antimicrobial activity for this compound.

It should be noted that the addition of unsaturation to a fatty acid greater than C12 makes it more active. From our contemporary perspective, a clearer picture is emerging of the structure-function relationships with regard to the antimicrobial properties of fatty acids. The term "antimicrobial" denotes not only antibacterial effects but also antifungal/yeast and antiviral properties. It has been shown that enveloped viruses (herpes, etc.) in particular can also be inactivated by treatment with specific fatty acids. Envelope viruses possess lipid bilayers (envelopes) that surround the protein/nucleic acid of the virus. Chain length of carbon atom and the kind of unsaturation and geometric structure (cis, kinked chain versus trans, straight chain) are all-important to biological activity of lipids, as previously mentioned.

TABLE 3.1

Minimal Inhibitory Concentrations (mM) of Saturated and Unsaturated Fatty Acids

Fatty acid	Staphylococcus aureus	Streptococcus group A	Candida albicans
Caproic (C6:0)	NI	NI	NI
Caprylic (C8:0)	NI	NI	NI
Capric (C10:0)	2.90	1.45	2.49
Lauric (C12:0)	2.49	0.12	2.90
Myristic (C14:0)	4.37	0.55	4.37
Myristoleic (C14:1)	*0.44*	*0.11*	*0.55*
Palmitic (C16:0)	NI	3.90	NI
Palmitoleic (C16:1)	*0.98*	*0.10*	*0.49*
Stearic (C18:0)	NI	NI	NI
Oleic (C18:1 cis)	*NI*	*1.77*	*NI*
Elaidic (trans oleic)	*NI*	*NI*	*NI*
Linoleic (C18:2ω6)	*NI*	*0.09*	*0.46*
Linolenic C18:3ω3)	*1.79*	*0.35*	*NI*
Linolelaidic (trans linolenic)	*NI*	*NI*	*NI*
Arachidonic (20:4ω6)	*NI*	*NI*	*NI*

Acids in italics are unsaturated.

NI: Not inhibitory at the concentrations tested (1.0 mg/ml).

Note: Most gram-negative bacteria are not affected.

When plants or animals make unsaturated fats, they mostly build the kinked "cis" form. However, food manufacturers discovered that bubbling hydrogen through polyunsaturated oils creates "partially hydrogenated" fats that are less vulnerable to becoming rancid than the original oils and therefore have a longer shelf life.

This hydrogenation process converts the bent oleic "cis" form to a straightened "trans" form (see diagrams).

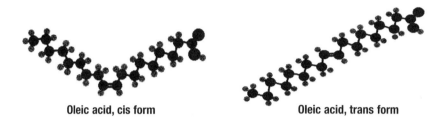

Oleic acid, cis form   Oleic acid, trans form

The chemical composition of the two forms is the same. The molecules have the same number of carbon, oxygen, and hydrogen atoms, the same COOH acid at the alpha end, and the double bond in the same place—but one is straight instead of kinked. Even though it is still unsaturated, the trans fats behave like saturated fats. There is presently a "trans hysteria" promulgated in many articles in technical journals, magazines, and newspapers that trans fats are more hypercholesterolemic than saturated fats. Trans fats have been used for several decades without so much alarm about their nutritional hazard to consumers. Whether trans fats are a real health problem in a **balanced** diet remains to be proven.

The body recognizes this trans chemical structure and tries to use it in the same places and for the same purposes that it uses the bent cis form. But the trans form stacks together just like saturated fats, which sabotages the flexible, porous functionality the cell needs from unsaturates.

In regard to the chemical chain configuration, certain generalizations can be made concerning the effect of these fatty acids on any microorganism. The cis form of a fatty acid is an active biocide, while the trans form of the same fatty acid is inactive. Medium-chain saturated fatty acids have killing effects preferably against gram-positive bacteria, while gram-negative bacteria are less affected. Shorter-chain (i.e., <C8, C10 carbon atoms) fatty acids inhibit gram-negative bacteria and fungi/yeast, and to a lesser degree gram-positive bacteria. As a compromise, lauric acid (C12) was found to be the most active saturated fatty acid against most microorganisms.

Monoglycerides as Antimicrobial Agents

My own research was the first report to show that the addition (esterification) of fatty acids to a monohydric (having a single OH group) alcohol, such as methanol or ethanol, reduced or eliminated the antimicrobial activity of fatty acids. The addition of a fatty acid to a polyhydric (more than one OH group) alcohol, however, produces a monoglyceride that is much more antimicrobial than the fatty acid alone (Kabara, Swieczkowski, et al., 1972).

Monoglycerides are widely used in foods, cosmetics, and pharmaceuticals as emulsifiers (substances that allow oil and water to be combined into a stable system without separation). In the past, the most important member of this group was glycerol monostearate (GMS). Many different grades of this emulsifier are available. They vary in purity of stearic acid used and generally are a mixture of mono-, di-, and triglycerides. The usual commercial-grade GMS and other commercial monoglycerides have a monoester content of only 40–45%. The more highly purified distilled monoglycerides (>90% monoester content) similar to Lauricidin behave differently than the usual grade of GMS. Emulsions made with highly purified GMS have smaller and more even particle size, which results in a more stable system. Uniform, stable emulsions are easier to preserve than unstable systems. Specific monoglycerides such as glycerol monolaurate (Lauricidin) are antimicrobial, while even pure GMS is not antimicrobial.

In other words, while certain fatty acids are antimicrobial, their combination with a monohydric alcohol (e.g. methanol and ethanol) results in a chemical form that is inactive. My research indicated, however, that the same reaction with polyhydric alcohol (glycerol, sugar, etc.) forms an ester that is an active product. Glycerol, one of the more common polyhydric (more than one OH group) alcohols, was esterified and the ester form was found to be more active than the corresponding fatty acids. I published extensive details of these findings. (See Reference list B, the volumes published by The American Oil Chemists' Society, *The Pharmacological Effect of Lipids*, Vol. I, Ch. 1 (1978), Kabara, J.J., "Fatty Acids and Derivatives as Antimicrobial Agents—A Review.")

Many other investigators have independently confirmed our initial findings. Reports by both Beuchat and Shibasaki confirmed the findings that Lauricidin is the most active of a series of monoglycerides, even in the presence of other foodstuffs (Beuchat 1980; Shibasaki and Kato in *The Pharmacological Effect of Lipids*, Vol. I, Ch. 2, 1978). Beuchat compared the effects of glycerol and sucrose esters, benzoate, sorbic acid, and potassium sorbate against *Vibrio parahaemolyticus* and found that the C12 monoglyceride (Lauricidin a.k.a. monolaurin) was more active than lower- or higher-chain-length derivatives. In addition, the low minimum inhibitory concentration value using monolaurin (5 ppm) showed it to be more effective than sodium benzoate (≥300 ppm) or even the much used food preservative sorbic acid (70 ppm). Because these esters are generally regarded as inactive against gram-negative bacteria, the inhibition of *V. parahaemolyticus* growth was somewhat surprising, although Shibasaki and Kato (1978) did report inactivating effects on a gram-negative bacterium. In these special cases, the Japanese researchers demonstrated that compounds that surround metal ions (chelating agents, such as citric, lactic, and polyphosphoric acid) are necessary to have an enhancing effect on the antibacterial action of monoglycerides against gram-negative bacteria.

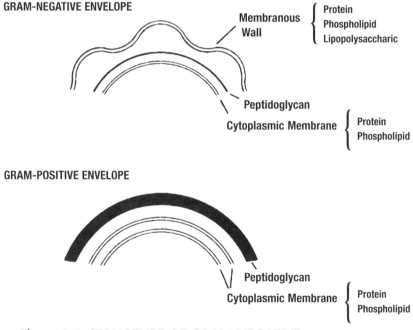

Figure 3.1: STRUCTURE OF GRAM-NEGATIVE AND GRAM-POSITIVE BACTERIA

Chelating agents are known to remove the outer membranous layer of the gram-negative bacteria (see Fig. 3.1) and enable preservatives and antibiotics to act on the bacteria as if it were a gram-positive specie. It should be noted, however, that the presence of added chelating agents is not always a prerequisite for demonstrating an inhibitory action of monoglycerides against gram-negative bacteria. As stated earlier, Beuchat observed that certain monoesters even without a chelating agent still adversely affected *V. parahaemolyticus* in a manner similar to that of gram-positive bacteria.

The antimicrobial activity of monoesters of glycerol (monoglycerides) compare favorably in activity with commonly used food preservatives such as parabens, sorbic acid, and dehydroacetic acid (Tables 3.2 and 3.3). The smaller minimum inhibitory concentration numbers in the table mean greater antimicrobial activity.

TABLE 3.2

Comparison of Antifungal Activities of Fatty Acid Esters with Some Commonly Used Preservatives

Minimum inhibitory concentration (ppm)			
Food preservatives	**Aspergillus niger**	**Candida utilis**	**Saccharomyces cerevisiae**
Monocaprin	123	123	123
Monolaurin (Lauricidin)	137	69	137
Butyl-p-hydroxybenzoate	200	200	200
Sodium lauryl sulfate	100	400	100
Sorbic acid	1000	1000	1000
Dehydroacetic acid	100	200	200

TABLE 3.3

Comparison of Antibacterial Activities of Fatty Acid Esters
with Some Commonly Used Preservatives

	Minimum inhibitory concentration (ppm)		
Food preservatives	**Bacillus subtilis**	**Bacillus cereus**	**Staphylococcus aureus**
Monocaprin	123	123	123
Lauricidin	17	17	17
Butyl-p-hydroxybenzoate	400	200	200
Sodium lauryl sulfate	100	100	50
Sorbic acid	4000	4000	4000

Antiviral Effects of Fatty Acids and Monoglycerides

Three lipid-containing bacterial viruses have been characterized in some detail in recent years. (A bacteria that is infected with a virus used for research is called a bacteriophage.) Three bacteriophages—PM2, Ø6, and PR4—were used to carry out a comprehensive survey of the potential antiviral properties of fatty acids and mono-, di-, and triglyceride derivatives (Sands et al. in *The Pharmacological Effect of Lipids,* Vol. I, Ch. 8, 1978). Fatty acids of chain length from 6 to 20 carbon atoms and various degrees of unsaturation were tested for antiviral activity. The effects on (a) virus inactivation, (b) inhibition of virus replication, and (c) any inhibition of cell growth by the agents were determined. In many cases of antiviral activity, concentration of the lipids was below 50 µg/ml or 50 ppm. At low concentrations, rarely were any deleterious effects on the growth of the bacterial host cells detected.

The inactivation of these phages (bacterial viruses) and the envelope Herpes virus by monoglycerides is presented in Table 3.4.

TABLE 3.4

Inactivation of Herpes Simplex Type 2 and Bacterial Phages by Monoglycerides

Monoglyceride	Concentration (ppm) giving 50% Survival*		
	HSV-2	Ø6	PM2
Lauricidin (C12)	12.5	10	10
Monopalmitin (C16)	>25	10	>25
Monopalmitolein (C16:1)	0.62	0.5	10
Monostearin (C18)	>25	>25	>25
Monoolein (C18:1)	0.16	0.5	5

*Virus suspensions exposed to monoglycerides for 30 minutes at 25°C.

It is important to note that nonlipid-containing phages PR4, T4, and Ø23 were not inactivated in vitro by any of these agents at low concentrations. Although low concentrations of monoglycerides do not inactivate phage PR4, the replication of this virus is inhibited by a variety of these agents, but only at higher (>50 ppm) concentrations.

Studies also show that HSV-2, a lipid virus associated with genital herpes, is inactivated by many of the same lipid agents that are active against the phages. The results indicate that Lauricidin (monolaurin) is a potent inactivator of HSV-2. The active saturated monoglyceride, Lauricidin, is now being taken for human herpes viral problems. Present clinical experience indicates that Lauricidin is a superior suppressor of Herpes viral outbreaks, even when compared to antiviral drugs. (See the Testimonials section, Chapter 13.)

The early stage of the infectious process is inhibited by fatty acids and monoglycerides. This suggests that the inhibited stage might be at the entry (membrane effects) process. One indication of successful entry (and subsequent viral genome expression) by the virus is the death of the host cell. The loss of cellular colony-forming ability due to virus infection was assayed in the presence and absence of fatty acids. The results showed that in the presence of lauric acid/monolaurin, the killing of the host cells by the virus is prevented (Isaacs and Thormar 1995).

Electron microscope studies indicate that the first stages of the viral replication process probably involve initial virus binding to the cell membrane and reorientational motion of the virus on the membrane to achieve proper positioning for entry. The presence of fatty acid suggests that fusion between the cell surface membrane and the virus membrane might occur during entry to allow the deposition of the virus DNA into the cell. Fatty acids seem to inhibit this entry and enhance the release of virus components from the cell surface.

Many of the agents active against various bacteria, yeast, and fungi studied in our laboratory were also found to be similarly effective against lipid-containing viruses. Thus, certain fatty acids and particularly their monoglyceride ester like monolaurin have wide-spectrum activity against a variety of microorganisms.

TABLE 3.5

Examples of Microorganisms Inactivated by Lauricidin

VIRUSES

HIV or HIV-1, -6	Visna virus
Herpes simplex virus-i (HSV-1 &2)	Vesicular stomatitis virus (VSV)
Measles virus	Rubella virus
Epstein-Barr virus	Respiratory syncytial virus
Influenza virus	Dengue virus (Type 1–4)
Leukemia virus	Cytomegalovirus (CMV)
Semliki forest virus	Lymphocytic choriomeningitis
Human papilloma virus (HPV)	Pneumovirus

BACTERIA

Gram-positive organisms

Bacillus anthracis (Anthrax)	Listeria monocytogenes
Staphylococcus aureus	Groups A, B, F, & G streptococci
Streptococcus agalactiae	Mycobacteria
Clostridium perfringens	

Gram-negative organisms

Chlamydia pneumonia	Neisseria gonorrhoeae
Helicobacter pylorus	Mycoplasma pneumonia
Vibrio parahaemolyticus	
Others if used concurrently with a chelator	

Fungi/Yeasts and Molds

Aspergillus niger	Saccharomyces cerevisiae
Penicillium citrinum	Ringworm or tinea (Trichophyton)
Candida utilis	Malassezia, species

A number of protozoa like *Giardia lamblia* are also inactivated or killed by Lauricidin (monolaurin).

Mode of Action of Fatty Acids

The antimicrobial properties of fatty acids have been investigated using a diverse array of organisms and methodologies. However, information on the mechanism of fatty acid interference with cell activity is scarce. Less is known about direct interference with cellular protein or nucleic acid synthesis. Also, the mechanism of saturated fatty acids appears to be different from that of polyunsaturated fatty acids.

The undissociated form of the fatty acid (COOH, not the dissociated salt form COO-) is responsible for antimicrobial activity, and therefore pH determines the extent of this dissociation. In the more basic or alkaline (pH>7.0) media, the salt form is more prominent and therefore the fatty acid is less active. Short-chain fatty acids are generally toxic to bacteria at relatively high concentrations and are known to have an adverse effect on the energy metabolism of a wide variety of microorganisms. Polyunsaturated long-chain fatty acids are different and affect specific groups of bacteria by mechanisms distinct from their saturated counterparts. In addition to direct interaction with the cell membrane (as with saturated fatty acids), polyunsaturated fatty acids may inhibit by other mechanisms. Polyunsaturated fatty acids exert some antimicrobial activity through auto-oxidation by the formation of active peroxides and other oxygen metabolites. The toxicity of linoleic acid, for instance, is attributed to the formation of short-chain aldehyde compounds by auto-oxidation. These oxygen metabolites, including peroxides, super oxide anions, and singlet oxygen, are all toxic to bacteria but also unfortunately to cells of the host.

Hence, short-chain saturated fatty acids and long-chain polyunsaturated fatty acids appear to exert their antimicrobial effects by different mechanisms.

The molecular structures of active fatty acids must relate to their ability to react with the cell membrane. It can be speculated that the tail of a fatty acid (hydrocarbon chain, C_{H3}-C_{H2}-C_{H2}-C_{H2}-) is inserted into the bilayer of the cell outer membrane, which then destabilizes the membrane. Membrane destabilization differs with fatty acids of dissimilar chain length and unsaturation. This destabilization results in increased membrane fluidity and alters vital membrane-associated functions such as aggregation, fusion, and permeability.

Even small concentrations of certain fatty acids have been found to inactivate enzymes in outer membranes. It is generally proposed that fatty acid regulation of sodium channels is mediated by its effect on membrane fluidity. The precise mechanism by which fatty acids affect ion channels remains to be discovered.

Fatty acids also can inhibit various enzymatic activities of bacteria, especially those of membrane-associated enzymes. There are two possible mechanisms, the first being indirect inhibition resulting from structural changes of the cell membrane, and the second involving direct reaction with enzyme proteins. Both mechanisms have been shown to be possible. Sheu and Freese (1972) considered that fatty acids may reversibly react with membrane proteins, altering the structure or uncoupling the electron transport chain having to do with energy of the cell.

Fatty acids are also known to have metabolic regulatory roles in the intercellular cytoplasm. Fatty acids may play a regulatory role in the spore formation of *B. subtilis.* At critical concentrations, fatty acids act as a signal for the initiation of sporulation (the method by which some bacteria multiply). The effective level may be an indicator of membrane synthesis or specific membrane-associated activities. Being integral components of other membrane lipids, fatty acids may serve to sense perturbations of membrane-associated metabolic events and cause a microorganism to protect itself by a spore form. Spores are very resistant to antibacterial agents.

Fatty acids may also act as signal messengers, transmitting environmental or metabolic information to components of a metabolic pathway. Our original research (Kabara et al.) demonstrated that added cis-unsaturated acids disorder the lipid hydrocarbon chains in lipid bilayers of a cell, but trans-unsaturated or long-chain saturated fatty acids have little or no effect. This difference in structure-function activity has been previously identified for fatty acids as antibacterial agents. Such observations confirm the explanation that the cell membranes are the primary site of action by fatty acids. Fortunately our body cell membranes are sufficiently dissimilar from microorganisms and are not affected by the fatty acids in the same manner. Hence, fatty acids are non-toxic.

Mode of Action of Monoglycerides

Research reveals that the inhibition activity of monoglycerides against amino acid transport in bacterial cells is due to interference with coupling of energy. The studies further observed that these antibacterial agents at bacteriostatic concentrations (growth inhibition, not killing) produce both stimulation of oxygen uptake and inhibition of energy-dependent amino acid transport (Scholz et al. 1984).

Another mechanism of action can be proposed from the fact that monoglycerides are known to decrease glycolysis (the enzymatic breakdown of compounds and subsequent release of energy) and to stimulate the production of glucose by the liver from substances other than carbohydrates—for example, proteins and fats. Glycolytic compounds like glucose and fructose reduce the growth inhibition of *B. subtilis* by monoglycerides (i.e., the bactericidal effect is not as strong with sugars as it is with fats). Tsuchido et al. (1987) found that autolysis of *B. subtilis* cells was induced by glycerol and sucrose esters of fatty acids. They demonstrated that these esters cause morphological changes in cells, suggesting that inhibition of some processes of synthesis or regulation of the cell membrane is related to the induction of autolysis.

Oleic acid does not alter the susceptibility of *M. pneumoniae* to antibiotics like erythromycin or tetracycline. In stark contrast, monoolein, the monoglyceride, increased *M. pneumoniae* susceptibility to the antibiotic tetracycline. This combination indicates that monoglycerides like monoolein and monolaurin affect membrane permeability. This theory is supported by the study of Muranushi et al. (1981), who demonstrated that monoolein enhances the permeability of artificial lipid membranes. Such studies show that the effects of monoglycerides are different from those of free fatty acids.

Studies in the past decade support the hypothesis that mycoplasma cells have receptors on their surface to attract monoglycerides. If this is true, it is possible that certain monoglycerides such as monolaurin (Lauricidin) attach to these receptor sites without being incorporated into the membrane. At partially inhibitory concentrations, the antibiotic tetracycline and active monoglycerides showed a synergistic effect. Tetracycline alone (0.1 ppm) produced no *M. pneumoniae* growth inhibition, nor did 25 or 50 ppm of monoolein; however, combinations at these concentrations produced 22% inhibition. Subcultures of these combination-treated cultures showed no viability, whereas viability was detected in subcultures of *M. pneumoniae* treated separately with 0.3 ppm tetracycline or with 75 ppm monoolein.

These results indicate that monoglycerides and antibiotics in combination would be more effective in treating patients with *M. pneumoniae* than antibiotic alone. Pertaining to this therapeutic approach with monoglycerides like monolaurin, ***concentrations of antibiotics employed could be lowered, and the development of resistance might be retarded or even averted.*** Certainly any drug side effects of the antibiotics would be reduced.

A more complete discussion on resistant organisms follows in the next chapter.

CHAPTER 4

Antimicrobial Activity and Resistant Organisms

Ever since antibiotics became widely available in the 1940s, they have been hailed as miracle drugs able to eliminate germs. Yet with each passing decade, microorganisms appear that defy not only single but multiple antibiotics.

People should realize that although antibiotics are needed to control microbial infections, they also have broad, undesirable effects on microbial ecology. That is, they can produce long-lasting change in the kinds and proportions of bacteria colonies—and the mix of antibiotic-resistant and antibiotic-susceptible types—not only in the treated individual but also in the environment. Antibiotics should therefore be used only when they are truly needed. For instance, they should not be administered for viral infections, for which they have no success in treating. The wide use of antibiotics in animal feed has led to a subsequent increase of resistance to them. This practice should not only be discouraged but outlawed. In this regard Lauricidin or other form of monolaurin supplementation may be a safe and effective alternative.

The antibiotic resistance problem is significant. More than 50 million pounds of antibiotics are produced each year in the U.S., and about 40% of that is used in livestock, mostly for growth promotion.

Nearly 80% of farm animals—mainly cattle, pigs, and poultry—receive subtherapeutic levels of antibiotics in their feed, at least part of the time. The use of such low levels has led to an increase in microorganism resistance to these antibiotics. Resistance by microorganisms that cause disease in humans and animals has risen sharply over the past several decades, not only in the U.S. but also in much of the world. Evidence is rapidly accumulating that this resistance is primarily promoted by the low levels of antibiotics given routinely to livestock.

The Challenge of Antibiotic Resistance

Today bacterial infections now defy most antibiotics. Worldwide, many strains of *Staphylococcus aureus* (approximately 93%) are already resistant to penicillin and methicillin but not to vancomycin. However, in a 1999 report *S. aureus,* an often-deadly bacterium, even responded poorly to vancomycin in three geographically separate patients. Emergence of forms lacking sensitivity to vancomycin signifies that variants untreatable by every known antibiotic are becoming more prevalent. *S. aureus,* a major cause of hospital-acquired infections, has thus moved one step closer to becoming an unstoppable killer. Fortunately, the *Staphylococcus* microbe is still susceptible to other drugs. However, the appearance of *S. aureus* not readily cleared by vancomycin is yet another indication of current (and looming) trouble resulting from the misuse of germicides.

The extensive irresponsible exploitation of antibiotics in medicine, animal care, and agriculture constantly selects for strains of bacteria that become resistant to antibiotics. If germicides are to retain their effectiveness over pathogens, they have to be used less often and more sensibly.

Bacteria can acquire resistance genes through several different routes. Many inherit the genes from their forerunners. Other times genetic mutations, which occur readily in bacteria, will spontaneously produce a new resistance trait or will strengthen an existing one. Frequently, bacteria will gain a defense against an antibiotic by taking up resistance genes from other bacterial cells in the vicinity. Thus bacteria may acquire resistance to a given drug by mutation of pre-existing genes or by the acquisition of new genes from other bacteria.

Resistance genes are commonly carried on plasmids, tiny loops of DNA that help bacteria survive various hazards in the environment. The genes may also occur on the bacterial chromosome, the larger DNA molecule that stores the genes needed for the reproduction and routine maintenance of a bacterial cell.

Often one bacterium will pass resistance traits to others by giving them a useful plasmid for their protection. Even viruses play a role in bacterial resistance. Viruses can extract a gene from one resistant bacterial cell and inject it into a different one. In addition, after a bacterium dies and releases its contents into the environment, another will occasionally take up for itself a liberated gene that gives resistance to the recipient bacteria.

As discussed above, the evolution and spread of bacteria resistant to beta-lactam (ß-lactam) antibiotics like penicillin has progressed at an alarming rate. Evolution is often thought of as occurring over a long time frame. However, the evolution of antibiotic resistance in bacteria can and does occur in a relatively short period, as the development of resistance to ß-lactam antibiotics demonstrates.

ß-lactam antibiotics, such as penicillin and cephalosporin as well as methicillin, ampicillin, and amoxicillin, are among the most frequently used antimicrobial agents. Bacteria never exposed before to penicillin protect themselves by producing a new enzyme, ß-lactamase, which degrades the antibiotic. How smart is that? This is how these simple organisms evolve mechanisms of resistance to ß-lactam antibiotics. This enzyme cleaves part of the structure in the ß-lactam ring of the antibiotic, rendering such antibiotics harmless to the bacteria. Thus the enzyme, ß-lactamase, confers upon pathogenic bacteria a resistance to lactam antibiotics. The genes programming for ß-lactamase production are found on the bacterial chromosome or on plasmids. Thus, the presence of resistant genes in plasmids and other transposable elements allows the genes to be transferred to other, even distantly related bacteria. You can see how antibiotic resistance represents a serious threat to effective clinical antimicrobial therapy.

As an example, antimicrobial resistance for lower respiratory tract infections has dramatically increased in the United States. Nearly all clinical isolates of *Moraxella catarrhalis* now produce the enzyme ß-lactamase. A linear increase in the prevalence of ß-lactamase-mediated ampicillin resistance has also been evident among isolates of *Haemophilus influenza* during the past decade (1995 to 2005). By the next decade, 50–60% of isolates of this organism are likely to produce ß-lactamase and become resistant. Although the susceptibility of this organism to alternative oral antimicrobials varies, rates of resistance to other non ß-lactam antibiotics remain less than 1% (fortunately). The rate of penicillin resistance among isolates of *Streptococcus pneumoniae* has also increased steadily in recent years and will likely reach 40–50% by 2012 if not sooner (Mera 2005). Because of cross-resistance, all ß-lactam antimicrobials now have reduced effectiveness in killing bacteria.

Resistance even occurs with germicides used in hand-washing products (Barry et al. 1984). During a 1984 investigation in a surgical intensive care unit, several bottles of the antiseptic hand-washing soap, OR [Operating Room] Scrub, were found contaminated with *Serratia marcescens*. The OR Scrub contained 1% of the common biocide triclosan. The antimicrobial efficacy of OR Scrub was examined *in vitro* using serial two-fold dilution method. The soap solution was inoculated with various concentrations of different nosocomial pathogens (meaning those that originate or occur in a hospital). The minimal bactericidal concentration of OR Scrub against *Pseudomonas aeruginosa* and several strains of *S. marcescens* was found to be less than or equal to a dilution ratio of 1:2. This means that any dilution of the OR Scrub solution greater than 1:2 would be ineffective. By comparison, a non-antiseptic soap from the same manufacturer (Wash) had a minimal bactericidal concentration for all strains tested at a dilution of at least 1:4. This was the first report of extrinsic contamination of antiseptic soap containing triclosan. No infections, however, could be attributed to the contaminated soap, but sporadic outbreaks of *Serratia* have occurred in this particular intensive care unit with no identifiable source. Although there have been few reported studies on the impact of antiseptic soap in reducing nosocomial infection, we question whether a soap with the limitations of OR Scrub should be used in intensive care units or operating rooms. Since this initial finding in 1984, more reports continue to be published indicating resistance to triclosan, which is omnipresent in so many antibacterial household products.

Easily incorporated into liquids, fabrics, and solid surfaces, triclosan's use has soared since its introduction in 1970. Scientists once believed that bacteria couldn't develop resistance to triclosan because it acts more like a grenade than a bullet. They thought the antiseptic killed bacteria in multiple ways rather than targeting a single protein/enzyme, the modus operandi of most antibiotics.

In the past few years, however, biologists have discovered that triclosan's main method of killing is very specific. It inhibits an enzyme involved in fatty acid synthesis. It has also been shown that some bacteria with mutations in that enzyme's gene can resist triclosan. More troubling, an antibiotic commonly employed against the tuberculosis bacterium targets the same enzyme, raising the possibility that triclosan use will lead to new antibiotic-resistant strains of the microbe.

Each reported study on triclosan-resistant microbes raises concern that the antiseptic's increasing popularity will encourage the evolution of bacteria impervious to drugs. For the moment, however, that worry remains theoretical, although the well-documented trend of accelerating rates of resistance is more than theoretical (Suller and Russell 2000).

Saturated Fatty Acids and Medium-Chain Monoglycerides: An Alternative Antimicrobial Agent

Now let us turn to the future of medium-chain fatty acids and their corresponding glycerol derivatives (like monolaurin) as antimicrobial agents. Will they become part of the solution for drug resistance or part of the problem? Present data based on these types of lipid antimicrobial agents suggest that high-quality monolaurin such as Lauricidin will be an answer not only ***because it does not form resistant organisms,*** but because it helps other antibiotics overcome resistance. In other words, the metabolic effect of certain fatty acids may improve the killing effect of antibiotics in the body.

In initial testing of clinical *Staphylococcus aureus* isolates with varying degrees of resistance to usual antibiotics, the minimum inhibitory concentration values for Lauricidin were all identical. (This is my line of research I am discussing now.) This was an early (1966) observation that organisms resistant to antibiotics showed no similar effects when our specially prepared high-quality monolaurin was used. Our initial findings were confirmed and expanded upon by Kitahara et al. (2004). Saturated fatty acids also show the identical minimum inhibitory (MIC) values across the board (see Table 4.1).

TABLE 4.1

Minimum Inhibitory Concentration (MIC) Values (ppm, parts per million) of antimicrobial agents against Staphylococcus aureus

Antimicrobial Agents	MSSA	MRSA			
ATCC	29213	4952	6849	3818	352
Octanoic acid (C8)	>1600	>1600	>1600	>1600	>1600
Decanoic acid (C10)	800	800	800	800	800
Lauric acid (C12)	400	400	400	400	400
Myristic acid (C14)	1600	>1600	800	1600	>1600
Palmitic acid (C16)	>1600	>1600	>1600	>1600	>1600
Stearic acid (C18)	>1600	>1600	>1600	>1600	>1600
Oxacillin	~0.5	16	>16	16	>16
Ampicillin	2	16	>16	>16	>16
Cefpirome	1	4	4	4	>16
Minocycline	~0.5	~0.5	~0.5	~0.5	~0.5

MSSA= Methicillin-Susceptible Staphylococcus aureus
MRSA= Methicillin-Resistant Staphylococcus aureus
Each compound was measured three times.

It should be noted that the minimum inhibitory concentration values for individual fatty acids are essentially the same for MSSA and MRSA. This means that there is no difference in susceptibility between MSSA and MRSA organisms when exposed to saturated fatty acids. MIC values for MRSA with the antibiotic oxacillin increased thirty times or more over values for MSSA. Fortunately, minocycline is still an effective antibiotic—so far.

A paper on acne patients (Eady 1998) reported that an increase in the number of multiply-resistant (greater than three resistances) staphylococci occurred in 67% of tetracycline-treated and 33% of minocycline-treated patients by the end of the 24-week treatment period. So you see it is only a matter of time before even minocycline becomes less effective.

Lack of differences in MIC value of saturated fats between MSSA and MRSA organisms strongly indicates that antimicrobial lipids can overcome microorganisms' resistance, since all the isolates were resistant to most of the antibiotics but not to lauric acid. My extended experience allows me to include Lauricidin in this generalization since lauric acid and the monoglyceride have similar effects.

Most important and different from drug antibiotics is the fact that there appears to be very little development of resistance in organisms to the bactericidal effects of these natural antimicrobial lipids like monolaurin (Petschow et al. 1996).

Flournoy et al. (1985) found that a number (101) of oxacillin-resistant Staphylococci all had the same minimum inhibitory concentration and minimum bactericidal/kill concentration values to monolaurin. This indicates that resistance to monolaurin in this instance was also shown not to be a problem, even though the bacteria were all resistant to oxacillin (see Table 4.1).

In 1982, Nickerson, Kramer, and Kabara observed microbial growth in a sink containing 1% alconox, a popular antiseptic. The resistant microbes were identified as the gram-negative organism *Enterobacter cloacae*. This bacterium had previously been shown to be resistant to 10% benzalkonium chloride, a strong biocide. In our hands, *E. cloacae* was able to grow in the presence of 25% sodium dodecyl sulfate, 25% "Triton" X100, or 20% "Tween" 20, 40, 60 or 80 surfactants that usually can affect membranes of microorganisms and cause bacterial inactivation. Monolaurin alone had poor activity against this gram-negative organism. However, monolaurin was active at 0.5% when a chelating agent (0.1%) was added. It is now widely accepted that a chelating compound is necessary for most gram-negative organisms to be adversely affected by monolaurin.

Monolaurin was found to inhibit induction of resistance in *Enterococcus faecalis* by the antibiotic vancomycin (Ruzin and Novick 1998). Monolaurin suppressed the growth of vancomycin-resistant *Enterococcus faecalis* on petri plates with vancomycin. The induction of vancomycin resistance involves a membrane-associated signal transduction mechanism. In contrast, monolaurin has no effect on the induction of Erythromycin-inducible resistance in *S. aureus,* which does not involve membrane signal transduction. This tells us that monolaurin will prevent resistance to some antibiotics, but not all, depending on their mode of acquiring resistance. In any case, the use of monolaurin in antibiotic therapy is promising, either through preventing or overcoming resistance.

It was predicted from my earlier work with monolaurin that toxin production from *S. aureus* strains might be reduced by monolaurin. Schlievert et al. (1992) confirmed my prediction that concentrations below those inhibitory for growth would reduce toxin formation. These studies have shown that growth of *S. aureus* strains from patients with toxic shock syndrome and scalded skin syndrome was inhibited or delayed in the presence of 100 to 300 ppm of Lauricidin. This specific data confirmed earlier suggestions from our own laboratory that Lauricidin (monolaurin) would be effective in blocking or delaying the production of toxins by pathogenic gram-positive bacteria.

The greater effectiveness of monolaurin against antibiotic-resistant strains would also make it an important ingredient in antiseptic creams for topical application. This possibility assumes greater importance because of the sensitivity of antibiotic-resistant strains of *S. aureus* and *P. aeruginosa* that have been isolated from suppurative wounds (those that produce or discharge pus as a result of injury or infection).

Action of Dodecylglycerol

Another C12 saturated lipid that is similar to monolaurin and has been extensively studied is dodecylglycerol, an alkylglycerol. While lauric acid attached as glycerol forms an *ester,* monolaurin, the dodecylglycerol lipid, has an *ether linkage*. Ethers are a class of organic compounds in which two carbon-chain groups are linked by an oxygen atom, C-C—C—O-C-C-C-C. The more stable ether derivative, however, is not an approved food additive. Yet much of its biological action is similar or identical to that of monolaurin. (Ved et al. 1984) Therefore, biological effects measured for the ether form may reflect the same properties as the ester form. This allows us to speculate about further possible actions of monolaurin, based on the studies with dodecylglycerol. For example, the ether derivative dodecylglycerol has been found to be slightly more active than the ester against the bacteria *Streptococcus faecium.* As was shown by Kabara et al. (1972b) for the ester derivative (a.k.a. monolaurin), gram-positive bacteria are more susceptible to dodecylglycerol than are gram-negative bacteria.

Similar to monolaurin, the antibacterial action of dodecylglycerol is through a physical disturbance of the cell wall, as well as its ability to serve as an enzymatic effector. The autolysin activity (autolysin is an enzyme that can break down the cell in which it is produced) of whole cells of *S. faecium* was greatly increased by dodecylglycerol. The stimulation of autolytic activity and inhibition of cell growth respond in parallel to different concentrations of dodecylglycerol.

The dodecylglycerol has also been shown to inhibit the growth of members of two genera of yeasts, Candida and Cryptococcus. It is strongly synergistic with the antifungal amphotericin B. At one-half its MIC value (minimum inhibitory concentration), dodecylglycerol decreased the MIC of amphotericin B by as much as eighty-fold. This high degree of synergism between dodecylglycerol and amphotericin B was demonstrated against a number of species of yeasts including *Candida albicans, Candida tropicalis, Candida parapsilosis, Cryptococcus neoforrnans, Cryptococcus albidus,* and *Cryptococcus laurentii.*

This synergism with amphotericin B is promoted by increasing the interaction between membrane-bound ergosterol (a sterol similar to cholesterol) and amphotericin B. Meanwhile, it was found (Ved et al. 1990) that dodecylglycerol and penicillin G act synergistically to dramatically lower the minimum inhibitory concentration of each other on four gram-positive bacteria studied. At one-half its MIC, dodecylglycerol lowered the MIC of penicillin 50-fold. Under the same conditions, penicillin only lowered the MIC of dodecylglycerol 4- to 7.5-fold.

The synergy found in laboratory tests for combinations of antibiotics and monolaurin or dodecylglycerol needs to be more fully explored in clinical settings to determine the useful application of these *in vitro* findings. This could lead to nutritional support with monolaurin as an adjunct to antibiotic therapy in infectious disease states. This is especially needed to combat resistant strains like MRSA not normally affected by classical antibiotic/antifungal therapies.

In this regard, studies from the Mayo Clinic and 3M were recently reported on the increased resistance of *Staphylococcus aureus* to the antibiotic methicillin (Rouse, Rotger et al. 2005). Nasal carriage of methicillin-resistant *Staphylococcus aureus* (MRSA) by hospitalized patients has been associated with nosocomial transmission of MRSA. Nasal carriage is also recognized as a risk factor for *S. aureus* infection in patients with concomitant human immunodeficiency virus (HIV) infection, with intravascular devices, undergoing surgical procedures, on hemodialysis or continuous ambulatory peritoneal dialysis, or who have undergone liver transplantation. These studies concluded the following:

1. Treatment of *S. aureus* with methicillin in time produced resistant organisms, while the same exposure to lauric acid esters (including Lauricidin) did not. See Figure 4.1 on next page.

2. In animals colonized with *S. aureus* and decolonized with mupirocin, the results were 50%. A lauric ester composition or monolaurin decolonized 83% of the animals. Again this shows how the inclusion of a saturated fat like lauric acid or monolaurin into the diet prior and during antibiotic therapy could be beneficial in overcoming resistant organisms.

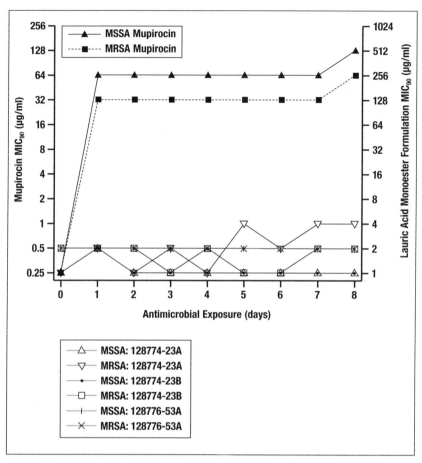

Figure 4.1

CHAPTER 5

Mother's Milk—The First Nutriceutical

It has long been suggested that breast-feeding gives the human infant a degree of protection from infectious illnesses—including gastroenteritis, otitis media (ear ache), and respiratory disease—that is not provided to infants ingesting cow's or synthetic milk. Modern studies confirm that human milk confers more advantages to babies against infectious agents, especially newborns in less than ideal conditions such as in many developing countries and under more bacteriological assault. Epidemiological investigations concerning the protective effects of human milk upon the infant have been conclusive. In countries where sanitary conditions are poor and infection rates are high, the incidence of bacterial infections is lowest in breast-fed infants.

Bacterial contamination of baby bottles and other feeding utensils is a major problem in poorer countries. Infants, of course, because of their natural susceptibility and the fact that some may be undernourished before supplementary feeding begins, are at the greatest risk from contaminated water used in food preparation and other dangerous environmental factors associated with poverty.

Of interest to our current discussion is the fact that mother's milk has high concentrations of palmitic acid, a saturated C16 fatty acid, and cholesterol. These are hardly poisons that nature would provide for the health of an infant.

I will describe how one special saturated lipid (monolaurin) of human milk is a unique protective factor for the infant.

Early Role of Mother's Milk as a Nutriceutical

It is accepted that human milk is rich in defense factors, including a growth enhancer of naturally beneficial bowel inhabitants such as lactobacilli, an anti-staphylococcal agent, immunoglobulins, certain complement components, Iysozyme, lactoperoxidase, lactoferrin and macrophages, lymphocytes, and lipids. Their proposed roles are given in the following table.

These listed factors protect both the mother's mammary gland and her infant from infection. Since the quantities of some of these factors are greater in human than in bovine milk, one would postulate that the resistance of breast-fed infants to infection would be superior to that of non-breast-fed infants. While there is no direct evidence that these defense factors are absorbed from the intestine of the infant, colostrum antibodies and lysozyme have been recovered from the stools of breast-fed infants. (Colostrum is the first milk produced by the breasts.) Colostrum provides a nursing infant with essential nutrients and infection-fighting antibodies. Furthermore, it appears that some of the factors remain active in the infant's intestine, making it more difficult for pathogenic microorganisms to colonize there.

TABLE 5.1

Host-Resistance Factors in Human Milk

Components

Protein Macromolecules	**Proposed Mode of Action**
Immunoglobulins ⟶	IgA for enhanced gut immunity
Complement: C3, C4 ⟶	C3 Fragments have opsonic, hemotactic, and anaphylatoxic activity
Lysozyme ⟶	Lysis of bacterial wall
Lactoperoxidase ⟶	Oxidation of streptococci
Lactoferrin ⟶	Binds iron needed by organisms

Humoral Factors

Leukocytes ⟶	Phagocytosis
Cell-mediated immunity ⟶	Production IgA, C4, and C3
Lactoferrin ⟶	Antimicrobial and immune booster
Polysaccharide Growth Factor for L. bifidus ⟶	Production of low pH that interferes with unwanted organisms' viability
Medium-Chain Lipids ⟶	Inactivation of bacteria, fungi, and viruses

As explained earlier, a nutriceutical is a functional food that has nutritional/caloric value in addition to pharmacological (drug) effects. Hippocrates (a Greek physician who lived circa 460–377 BC) recognized this truism when he declared in a famous aphorism, "Let thy food be your medicine and your medicine thy food." Historically, mother's milk must be considered the first nutriceutical. Mother's milk provides the infant with important nutrients for growth and development, and it also contains substances with antimicrobial and other protective properties.

This concept of human milk having sanitizing effects was recognized early in human medicine. In the history of cataract surgery, which extends back at least three thousand years, the translation of Hindu manuscripts gives detailed methods of the great surgeon Susruta. He described principles of surgery based on anatomic dissection. He practiced asepsis (fumigating the operating room with sweet vapors) and gave an excellent account of his technique of couching (depression of the lens into the vitreous fluid of the eye), as well as an outline of postoperative care. After couching, the milk of a nursing mother would be distributed into the eyes much in the way that antiseptics are now used after an operation.

Unfortunately, this knowledge was buried with the rise of the caste system of the Brahmins, who forbade dissection and the shedding of blood. The later rise of Buddhism may also have dampened the historical impact of early medical knowledge related to the Hindu religion. The surgeons gave way to the priests, and so the brilliant discoveries of the Hindus did not pass down to the Greeks or Egyptians. The knowledge that mother's milk acts as an antiseptic agent was lost until relatively recently, when a researcher found that cream but not skim milk was biologically active after standing (Fieldsteel 1974). Other studies of lipid properties found that certain fatty acids, in particular their monoglycerides, are antimicrobial. Tri- and diglycerides are *not* actively antimicrobial. Thus it was evident that the fat portion of human milk is biologically active because it is converted into two free fatty acids and a sn1(3)-monoglyceride (Kabara et al., circa 1966, published 1968).

When fresh samples of human and bovine milk were compared, the bovine samples were not antimicrobially active *in vitro*, even though both had similar fat/triglyceride content. This is because human milk contains a lipase enzyme that produces active fatty acids and monoglycerides from the milk fat upon standing. This is necessary since the human baby does not possess lipases at birth, while the calf does have lipase activity at birth. Thus human milk needs accompanying lipases from the mother to *predigest* the inactive fat (triglycerides) into active antimicrobial fatty acids and monoglycerides.

Antimicrobial Fatty Acids in Mother's Milk

Table 5.2 presents the antimicrobial activity of fatty acids found in mother's milk against some common microorganisms. (See also Welsh and May 1979, 1981; and Clarke and May 2000.)

Milk fatty acids also killed *Listeria monocytogenes* in a dose dependent manner, whereas much less killing of salmonella (a gramnegative organism) was observed (Sprong et al. 1999). The antimicrobial capacity of individual fatty acids depended on concentration and chain length.

The long chain saturated fatty acids C16:0 and C18:0, as well as the shorter-chain C4:0, C6:0, and C8:0, were not antimicrobial under these same concentrations.

Isaacs et al. (1991) added lipids—previously shown by Kabara et al. to have antiviral and antibacterial activity—to human milk, bovine milk, and infant formulas to determine whether increased protection from infection could be provided to infants as part of their diet. Again, saturated fatty acids with chain lengths varying from 8 to 12 carbons were found to be more strongly antiviral and antibacterial when added to milk than saturated long-chain (>C14) fatty acids. Since both cow's milk and artificial human milk are

TABLE 5.2

Minimal Inhibitory Concentrations (mM) of Fatty Acids
Found in Mother's Milk

Fatty acid	Staphylococcus aureus	Streptococcus Group A	Candida albicans
Capric (C10, 2.0%)*	2.90	1.45	2.90
Lauric (C12, 10%)	2.49	0.12	2.49
Myristic (C14, 6.0%)	4.37	0.55	4.37
Palmitic (C16, 22%)	NI	3.90	NI
Stearic (C18, 8.0%)	NI	NI	NI
Oleic (C18:1, 32%)	NI	1.77	NI
Linoleic (C18:2, 15%)	NI	0.09	0.46
Linolenic (C18:3, 0.1%)	1.79	0.35	NI

*Approximate concentration in mother's milk

NI = Not Inhibitory at the concentrations tested (1.0 mg/ml)

devoid of antimicrobial activity, such studies suggest that increased protection from infection could be provided to infants by the addition of antimicrobial medium-chain monoglycerides (such as monolaurin) to an infant's diet.

Antiviral Effects of Fatty Acids and Monoglycerides

While breast-feeding is important to the infant, transmission of the HIV-1 AIDS virus by infected mothers presents a big problem. Reducing HIV-1 transmission through breast milk would decrease the burden of pediatric HIV/AIDS. Microbiocidal treatment of expressed human breast milk infected with immunodeficiency virus type 1 (HIV-1) is a feasible option since an edible (i.e., non-toxic) acting agent is available (Lauricidin, the commercial form of monolaurin). In one report (Isaacs et al. 2006), breast milk from anonymous donors was artificially infected by adding cell-free and cell-associated HIV-1. The virucidal activity of lauric acid, C12, monolaurin (Lauricidin), monocaprin C, and 1-O-octyl glycerol (an ether of the C8 fatty acid) were tested. Virucidal activity was also tested against other enveloped (e.g. herpes simplex virus [HSV-2]) and non-enveloped (e.g. bovine papilloma virus [BPV-1]) viruses. All compounds had excellent to moderate overall virucidal activity. Monolaurin was one of the most effective against HIV-1. Thus, microbiocidal treatment of expressed human breast milk seems to be a feasible option to decrease the burden of pediatric HIV/AIDS.

My early attempts to interest several food companies in making better infant formulae by adding these active monoglycerides fell on non-responsive ears. This is an example of the NIH (Not Invented Here) syndrome (as opposed to the usual acronym for National Institutes of Health).

In addition to these antiviral effects, monolaurin is capable of inactivating other undesirable microorganisms, including fungi, several species of ringworm (Isaacs et al. 1995), and the yeast *Candida albicans* (Isaacs et al. 1991). The protozoan parasite *Giardia lamblia*, responsible for diarrhea in babies, is killed by monoglycerides from hydrolyzed human milk (Reiner et al. 1986; Crouch et al. 1991; Isaacs et al. 1995). *Chlamydia trachomatis* is also inactivated (Bergsson et al. 1998).

Chlamydia is the most common bacteria-related sexually transmitted disease in the United States. Current research involves development of a vaccine against *Chlamydia*. The problem, as with all vaccines, is that the vaccine being made needs to affect a wide range of different *Chlamydia* strains. Although this idea is not tested, I would advocate the daily addition of a monolaurin supplement rather than the present attempts to vaccinate young teenage girls.

Hydrogels containing monocaprin/monolaurin are potent *in vitro* inactivators of sexually transmitted viruses such as HSV-1 and HIV-2, and bacteria such as *Neisseria gonorrhea* and *Chlamydia trachomatis*.

TABLE 5.3

Viral inactivation by monoglycerides at 37°C (98°F) for 30 minutes

Monoglyceride	Concentration mg/ml(mM)	Reduction of virus titer ($\log_{10}$)	
		VSV[A]	HSV-1[A2]
Monocaprylin (8:0)[B]	2.0 (9)	>4.0	ND[C]
Monocaprin (10:0)	0.5 (2)	>4.0	3.7
Monolaurin (12:0)	0.25 (0.9)	>4.0	3.7
Monomyristin (14:0)	2.0 (13)	3.0	ND
Monoolein (18:1)	1.0 (2.8)	2.3	ND
Monolinolein (18:2)	0.25 (0.7)	>4.0	ND

[A] Vesicular stomatitis virus
[A2] Herpes simplex virus-1
[B] Carbon atoms: double bonds
[C] ND = Not Done

CHAPTER 6

Dietary Lipids in Oral Health

Tooth decay is the process that results in cavities (dental caries). It occurs when bacteria in your mouth, primarily *Streptococcus mutans,* make acids that eat away at the structure of the tooth. If not treated, tooth decay can cause tooth loss and gum disease. Bacterial infection of the tissues and bones that surround the teeth is called periodontal disease.

Periodontitis is an advanced form of gum disease in which the tissues and bones that support the teeth are damaged by the buildup of bacterial plaque. This plaque, also called dextran (a glucose polymer or polysaccharide), is produced by the action of *Strep. mutans* on sugar. This plaque becomes home to a whole host of other bacteria. If periodontitis is not treated, teeth can become loose and need to be removed or may fall out. Generally antibiotics are needed to help get rid of any infection. Dental infections can cause systemic problems that may even lead to heart disease. Emerging science suggests that there is a link between the health of your mouth and the health of your body. While physicians and dentists don't know the exact connection, several theories have been proposed. This will be discussed in Chapter 9.

The role of sugar and effects of protein malnutrition in dental caries seem to be well known. The place of fats or lipids in this dietary triumvirate of carbohydrate, protein, and fat, however, is less considered. Indeed, while the subject of dietary fat in heart disease is hotly debated in medical circles, the effect of fat on dental caries is largely ignored. Considering that the average diet contains 30–40% lipids, it seems incongruous that so little is known about the effects on our oral health of this dietary constituent that passes through the oral cavity in such abundance.

It is the purpose of this chapter to collate information on fats in relation to dental caries, and to show how monolaurin and certain saturated fatty acids can be useful for our oral and general health. The role of saturated fatty acids and monoglycerides on factors leading to dental decay will be examined from the point of view of their effects on other nutrients, and also their value as antimicrobial agents.

The Role of Lipids in Oral Biology

It is widely accepted that diet affects the lipid and fatty acid composition of teeth. Enamel and dentine structures reflect the composition of the diet, but to different extents. Because dietary lipids have such obvious effects on enamel and dentine, it would be of interest to know to what extent the change to a specific lipid composition during the weanling period might affect resistance to microorganisms as an adult. Such studies with specific lipids are only now being conducted.

A number of early investigators observed an association between high levels of dietary fat in certain populations and low incidence of dental caries. Strong interpretation of these findings is difficult because of the great disparity of dietary composition in other nutrients that could also influence caries. While it is difficult to isolate a cause-effect influence of fat on the caries process, earlier reports on the beneficial effects of fats were all but ignored by contemporary dental investigators.

Early investigators like Rosebury and Karshan (1939) studied the effects of oils and fats on caries. A 5% concentration of corn oil was more effective in reducing caries than 0.5% but not more effective than 2%. Cod liver oil was more effective than olive oil; paraffin oil, which is not a fat, was the least effective (i.e., does not metabolize to free fatty acids). In these cases, the effect is on microorganisms.

In another experiment, fat similar to that found in grain was added to the diet as free fat (in other words, as a separate ingredient). The two forms of the fat (one found naturally in the grain and the other simply added as free fat) were presumably equally utilizable in nutrition. However, a decrease in caries was found only in the added-fat group. **This means that the decrease in dental caries was likely exerted directly in the mouth by the fat rather than through nutritional or systemic channels.**

A literature review (Nizel 1969) examined the roles of fat, protein, and carbohydrate on dental caries. Not totally expected, the effects of fat in reducing caries appeared to be more pronounced than lowering carbohydrate levels. It was shown that both lard in the diet (primarily a saturated fat) and adequate protein levels are important in reducing caries.

The earliest animal studies (Aebi 1964) relating decreases in dental caries to increases in dietary fat were not conducted for that purpose. They were conducted to determine the effect of calcium, phosphorus, and vitamin D on the incidence of dental caries in rats. Oils were added to the dry diets of rats twice weekly. Dental caries incidence in the fissures of the rat teeth was reduced significantly by all three supplements. It was suggested that the added oil might have exerted a protective effect in the environment of the teeth rather than contributing to the mineralization process.

To separate the anticaries action of vitamin D from that of corn oil and to define more precisely the anticaries action of fats, a second series of experiments was carried out. This demonstrated that increasing concentrations of corn oil caused decreasing rates of dental caries. Caries were inhibited more in the rice diet than in the cornmeal diet at two concentrations of corn oil (2% and 5%). While the amount of total fat was higher in the cornmeal diet than in the rice diet, a higher reduction in dental caries was measured in the rice diet, which provided more free fat in the mouth than did the physically bound fat of the cornmeal. Olive oil, Wesson oil, Crisco, and lard were all found to inhibit caries as well as corn oil. The authors suggested that the oil-fat effect was a local one exerted in the mouth. They proposed that the fat may have lubricated the teeth or produced a film on either the food particles or the tooth surface. Either role could have prevented the bacterial digestion of food particles or the penetration of acid to the tooth surface.

In other studies (many have since been carried out), anticaries effect depended on the hardness or higher melting point of the various fats tested. Saturated fats have higher melting points. The greatest number of caries occurred with a fat-free diet, while the greatest decrease in caries was scored with hydrogenated oils (hard fat) with a melting point above body temperature. The currently fashionable fad for fat-free foods may not be best for our oral health.

While several investigations have demonstrated that caries can be inhibited by different kinds of fats, it would seem likely that coconut oil, which generates antimicrobial lipids (saturated medium-chain fatty acids and monoglycerides) in the mouth, would be even more effective than other oils in inhibiting caries. Unfortunately, there is no direct data supporting this hypothesis.

The Role of Lipids in Fluoride Metabolism

The role of fluoride in dental caries is well recognized. Fluoride toothpastes now account for 80–85% of the U.S. market and are becoming increasingly important in markets throughout the world. Fluoride content or concentration in the diet or dentifrice (or both) is not the sole criterion in predicting clinical effectiveness. The amount of "available" fluoride in these products determines how much is present to react with the teeth. Thus, any difference in effectiveness of fluoride in the diet or dentifrices in reducing dental caries may reflect factors that lower the amount of "free" or water-soluble fluoride available in the oral cavity or absorbed in the intestine.

This idea of bioavailability and not simply content or concentration of a constituent in a product has an extensive history in nutritional research. It is not what we eat that is important but rather what we absorb and the body uses. In the case of fluoride and dental caries, these two effects must be considered: activity on the teeth in the oral cavity, and whole body effects.

In the oral cavity, fluoride becomes incorporated into the dental enamel, thereby strengthening the teeth against acid attacks. Indirect inhibition effects on microorganisms cannot be excluded. Fluoride is a known inhibitor of several enzyme systems and has been shown to have antimicrobial action (though its mechanism of action in this latter respect is not certain).

Of greater interest and closer to the subject at hand is the influence of dietary fat on fluoride absorption. Rats were fed isoenergetic diets (same number of calories) with graded levels of fat (0, 10%, 30%, and 50%) containing 400 ppm fluoride. Tissue fluoride concentration increased as dietary fat increased. This was apparently caused by increased absorption of fluoride. Fluoride in the femur bone was increased and, without direct evidence, one can only speculate that fluoride uptake in teeth would also be increased.

Thus, the role of dietary fat in fluoride metabolism provides us with yet another alternative mechanism by which fat can influence dental caries: the more fat one eats, the better the body's uptake of fluoride (or so the theory and early evidence goes). One can speculate that fat and fluoride could have some beneficial preventive effects in relation to osteoporosis as well.

The Effect of Fatty Acids on Plaque Formation

It has been reported that the microorganisms causing pyorrhea (inflammation of the gums with a loosening of the teeth and a discharge of pus from the tooth sockets) could be successfully removed with a soap compound, sodium ricinoleate (salt of a fatty acid derived from castor oil). While sodium ricinoleate had little bactericidal qualities when tested (Sterling and Mead 1937), it lowered total oral bacterial growth for more than three hours in a mouthwash and dentifrice. The *in vivo* effectiveness of sodium ricinoleate was attributed more to the lipid's cleansing properties and peptizing action (helping in digestion of bacterial products) than to antibacterial action. The fatty acid cleansed the oral tissue so that less organic material remained to act as a culture medium for pathogenic organisms.

An early study by Schuster et al. (1980) demonstrated the effectiveness of certain fatty acids in reducing the acid dissolution of hydroxyapatite (inorganic constituent of bone). Saturated fatty acids with carbon chains numbering 8, 10, 12, 14, and 16 were tested. While saturated chain lengths C10 and C14 reduced acid formation compared to that observed in control tubes, saturated medium-chain C12 gave better than 50% reduction in acid as well as a reduction in microbial growth.

See the end of Chapter 13 for more details about the fatty acid as an ester called monolaurin (Lauricidin) and its effects on prevention of dental caries.

Oral Hygiene for the New Millennium

Data gathered as early as the 1930s indicated that the level of sugar is not the sole determining factor in cariogenesis (the development of dental caries, or cavities). It should be appreciated that sugar in foods does not exist as a separate entity; other nutrients (such as the quantity and type of protein in the diet and the quantity and type of fat) will and do affect the cariogenicity potential of the sugar. It must be recalled that experimental animals on a *well-balanced, nutritious* diet have low incidence of dental caries regardless of the sucrose concentration in their feed. This needs to be especially considered when giving high-sugar cereals/foods to children.

All high-sugar cariogenic diets cause deficient growth of animals as compared to their growth on ordinary laboratory chow. All cariogenic diets are very low in fat. Without belaboring the point, it should be obvious that the dietary intake of vitamins and minerals can also contribute in a positive manner to dental health. Therefore, any healthy diet should be considered as a complete system. A single component removed or added will disturb the system in many ways, and often in an unpredictable manner, unless the system's total combination of carbohydrate, protein, and fat is considered.

It should be noted that the food ingredients individually or in a processed food do not adequately define the absorbed composition of the diet. The interaction of food ingredients can increase or decrease their individual biological effects. In the case of sugar products, this sucrose content could actually lower the incidence of dental decay when combined with certain proteins, fats, etc. In other words, the level of sucrose *per se* in the product does not predict its cariogenic effect.

Until these and other questions can be answered clinically, it remains for animal experiments to provide us with dietary goals but not regulatory guidelines. Even here, caution is required in the interpretation of these animal models and their potential relevance to human conditions. It is worth repeating that dental infections can cause systemic problems that may lead to heart disease and other maladies. There is a link between the health of your mouth and the health of your body.

CHAPTER 7

Dietary Fat and the Immune System

Our immune system includes the skin, body organs, cells, cell products, and messenger molecules. This network of cells and messenger molecules communicates with each other. The immune system is designed to protect us from agents of disease and to heal wounds delivered by injury or invasion by microorganisms. In order to do its job properly, our immune system must be eminently sensitive in differentiating invaders (foreign) from our normal family members—our own native **self cells** and native **self molecules.** The immune system's task is to identify and then eliminate foreign (non-self) agents, be they bacteria, fungi, viruses, cancer cells, or toxic chemicals.

The basic concept of "self" and "non-self" is important to understand. During gestation of the fetus, the immune system recognizes all individual body cells and proteins as "self" or friendly; "non-self" are foreigners. At times after birth, the immune system can become dysfunctional and develop immune responses against the body's own proteins (and other molecules), resulting in autoimmunity. This same mechanism works against our own aberrant cells, which results in having tumor immunity. The present-day practice of routinely vaccinating infants with Hepatitis B should be discouraged because these antigens (vaccines) could be perceived by the body to be "self" proteins, and therefore lower amounts of antibody are formed later in life. Multiple simultaneous vaccines, especially when given to infants and very young children, may over-tax the immune system. I believe that the present system of multiple vaccinations to very young children causes more harm than good.

This chapter discusses how the immune system is affected by the kind (type) and especially the quantity of fat in the diet.

The complex human immune system is made up of a number of cell types and molecules that are scattered throughout the body. As shown in Table 7.1, there are two major parts: an innate and an adaptive immune response.

TABLE 7.1

The Human Immune System

Immune Response		
Innate	**Adaptive Mechanical Barrier**	
Immune cells	β-Lymphocytes	T-Lymphocytes
Macrophages	(Humoral	(Cell-Mediated
Neutrophils	Immunity)	Immunity)
Natural Killer (NK) Cells		

The innate system includes mechanical barriers and immune cells. The immune cells are composed of macrophages, neutrophils, and the natural killer (NK) cells. A "foreign" (non-self) aggressor activates the adaptive immune response.

Adaptive immunity includes two major categories of lympho-cytes, the cells that produce antibodies to specific foreign (non-self) agents: β-lymphocytes and T-lymphocytes. T-lymphocytes are so named because they pass from their bone marrow site of origin to the thymus (T) for maturation. β-lymphocytes are also generated in the bone marrow. Both may go to the peripheral lymphoid organs. For a complete discussion of the immune system, reviews on the subject by J.J. Pestka and M.F. Witt (1985) and John E. Upledger (2000) are highly recommended. The immune response may lead to disease (autoimmunity to self) as well as allergic reactions.

This chapter covers the differential effect of saturated and unsat-urated lipids on the immune response system. The immune sys-tem is affected by the kind of fat in the diet and even more so by high lipid levels. Therefore fats should not be labeled "bad" or even "good" since their ultimate biological effects depend on kind and quantity. Remember, it is not only *what you eat* that is important but also *how much* you eat.

Fatty Acids and the Immune Response

Research conducted with the cells of the immune system demon-strated two facts: First, the polyunsaturated essential fatty acids (EFAs) linoleic acid, or **omega-6,** and a-linolenic acid, or **omega-3,** are required for the growth and maintenance of these cells. Sec-ond, free (non-ester) fatty acids are produced and secreted during activation of the immune cells. Fatty acids at low concentrations stimulate several functions of the immune cells *in vitro*. High concentrations, however, are inhibitory. Review of the research on the subject has shown that at a given high concentration, polyunsaturated fats are more inhibitory than most saturated fats (Wanten and Calder 2007).

Animal studies have shown that both deficiency and excess of essential polyunsaturated fats can inhibit the immune response. The effect of omega-6 polyunsaturated fats (depending on concentration) ranged from no effect to inhibition, while that of omega-3 polyunsaturated fats ranged from inhibition to stimulation. Human epidemiological studies have also indicated possible links between fat intake and certain types of cancer, and the severity of autoimmune disorders. Thus, there are several lines of evidence suggesting that dietary fat may modulate an immune response in either a beneficial or a harmful direction for our body. Based upon such findings, studies have been conducted regarding the effects of total fat and its composition on the human immune response. Results from these studies are summarized below.

High-Fat Diets and the Immune Response

The influence of fats on the immune response in adult mice on one of the following four diets was recorded as follows: high polyunsaturated fatty acid, high saturated fatty acid, low polyunsaturated fatty acid, and a standard commercial diet (control). The three test-fat diets were designed to have approximately the same energy content, and the mice of each group maintained similar body weights. The high-fat diets significantly reduced the lymphocyte response to non-self antigens such as cancer cells. Tumor incidence was highest in rats with the least responsive lymphocytes, and lowest in rats with the most responsive lymphocytes. This points out that high-fat diets will increase the incidence of certain cancers (Doyle 2007).

Essential Fatty Acids and the Immune Response

The statement that essential fatty acids or EFAs—linoleic (18:2 omega-6) and a-linolenic (18:3 omega-3)—found in certain fats can affect the immune response is based on observations that EFA deficiency can accentuate or improve symptoms of certain autoimmune diseases in animals.

The effects of dietary fat on cell toxicity and antibody response are influenced by the fatty acid composition and amount of fat in the diet. High levels of dietary fat, particularly those containing polyunsaturated fatty acids, *suppress* lymphocyte function when EFA requirements are met but *intensify* these same responses in EFA deficiency; thus, dietary fats can differentially modulate the levels of lymphocyte T- and b-cell protection, depending on various dietary factors.

The influence on humoral immunity of a fat diet deficient in essential fatty acid and various levels of dietary polyunsaturated fatty acids indicates that:

1. Consumption of diets deficient in essential fatty acids (0% corn oil) significantly reduces the humoral immune response. This reduction was demonstrated after feeding an essential fatty acid-deficient diet for only 28 days. The reduced immune response

preceded any observable effects of essential fatty acid deficiency on growth or appearance.

2. After 56 days on this deficient diet, mice switched to the control diet (13% corn oil) for 7 days demonstrated full recovery of their humoral response.

3. These results support the hypothesis that the proper balance of essential fatty acids in fats plays a crucial role in maintaining the functional integrity of humoral immunity.

Ratio and Level of Polyunsaturated Fats in Relation to Lymphocyte Function

The effects of dietary polyunsaturated fatty acids upon blood lipid levels and lymphocyte functions were reviewed (Boissoneault et al. in Ching Kuang Chow, 1992). Diets differed in the ratio of omega-6 to omega-3 polyunsaturated fatty acids and in the absolute quantity consumed.

The results indicated that dietary alpha-linolenic acid (omega-3) has significant blood lipid-lowering and immunomodulatory effects, but that the effect is dependent upon the **total** polyunsaturated fatty acid content of the diet. The ratios of linoleic (omega-6) and alpha-linolenic (omega-3) acids to other fatty acids (e.g. saturated, monounsaturated omega-9) are crucial in determining the precise effect of manipulations of the fat composition of the diet. This is why a balance in dietary fat is so important for optimal health. When nutrients are available in a balanced way, the body is able to adjust to its needs.

The host response—a measure of cell-mediated immunity *in*

vivo—progressively decreased with increase in omega-3 polyunsaturated fatty acid. Alpha-linolenic acid from dietary fish oil (an omega-3 fat) results in lowered blood lipid levels and suppressed lymphocyte functions *in vitro* and *in vivo*. This means that while omega-3 has desirable effects in lowering blood lipids, it simultaneously weakens our immune system.

Numerous reports have shown that diets rich in omega-6 polyunsaturated fatty acid, as advocated by the American Heart Association, lead to significant negative changes for optimal health in regard to the metabolism of the immune tissues. Alterations of macrophage metabolism and function were examined in rats fed polyunsaturated or saturated fatty acid-rich diets. The polyunsaturated omega-6 group had *decreased* macrophage phagocytes such as white blood cells (which engulf and ingest non-self particles)—a change related to modifications of macrophage metabolism and a cause for increased tumor development. So while "saving" you from heart attacks, increased polyunsaturated fatty acids of the omega-6 variety makes you more prone to cancer.

The information that emerges is that too much (omega-6) or too little (omega-3) can be detrimental to good health. It needs to be emphasized that omega-6 and omega-3 compete for the same metabolic enzymes, thus the omega-6:omega-3 ratio will significantly influence the ratio of the ensuing eicosanoids (hormones—e.g. prostaglandins, leukotrienes, thromboxanes etc.) and will alter the body's metabolic function.

Metabolites of omega-6 are significantly more inflammatory (especially arachidonic acid) than metabolites from omega-3. This necessitates that omega-6 and omega-3 be consumed in a balanced proportion, with the ideal ratio of omega-6 to omega-3 ranging from 3:1 to 5:1. Studies suggest that the evolutionary human diet, rich in seafood, nuts, and other sources of omega-3, may have provided such a ratio.

Typical Western diets, however, provide ratios between 10:1 and 30:1—i.e., dramatically skewed toward omega-6. Here are the ratios of omega-6 to omega-3 fatty acids in some common oils: canola 2:1, soybean 7:1, olive 13:1, sunflower (no omega-3), flax 1:3, cottonseed (almost no omega-3), peanut (no omega-3), grape seed oil (almost no omega-3), and corn oil with a 46:1 ratio of omega-6s to omega-3s. It should be noted that olive, peanut, and canola oils consist of approximately 80% monounsaturated (C18:1, oleic acid) omega-9 fatty acids (i.e., neither omega-6 nor omega-3); thus they contain relatively small amounts of omega (3 and 6) fatty acids. Consequently, the omega-6 to omega-3 ratios for these oils (olive, canola, and peanut) are not as significant as they are for corn, soybean, and sunflower oils.

Obviously, we need both kinds but in a proper balance or ratio. This ideal ratio is probably 10–5:1 rather than the present 20:1 ratio found in most modern diets.

Some research has even shown that omega-3s help protect us from an array of illnesses. The benefits of omega-3s include reducing the risk of heart disease and stroke while helping to reduce symptoms of hypertension, depression, attention deficient disorder (ADD), joint pain and other rheumatoid problems, as well as certain skin ailments. Research indicates that omega-3s encourage the production of body chemicals that help control inflammation—in the joints, the bloodstream, and the tissues.

But just as important is omega-3's ability to reduce the negative impact of the other essential type of fatty acid, omega-6. Found in foods such as eggs, poultry, cereals, vegetable oils, baked goods, and margarine, omega-6s at some level are also considered essential. They support skin health, lower cholesterol, and help make our blood "sticky" so it is able to clot. However, when omega-6s aren't balanced with sufficient amounts of omega-3s, problems can ensue. Research indicates that high omega-6 fatty acids shift the physiologic state to pro-inflammatory.

Effect of Lipids on the Immune Response and Inflammation

To obtain further information about the effects of specific fatty acids, weanling male rats were fed saturated fats for six weeks on low-fat (7.7%) or high-fat (17.8%) diets, which differed according to the principal fatty acids present (see Ching Kuang Chow, editor). The diets were rich in caprylic (C8) and capric acids (C10) (medium-chain triglycerides, or MCTs), lauric acid, palmitic acid at the sn1(3) position of the monoglyceride, and palmitic acid or stearic acid at the sn2 position of glycerin. The total proportions of saturated (42–46%), omega-9 monounsaturated (36%), omega-6 polyunsaturated (15%), and omega-3 polyunsaturated (2.2%) fatty acids were the same in all diets.

The fatty acid composition of the blood serum and of spleen lymphocytes reflected the diet fed. Immune response was negatively affected by the high-fat diet: NK cell activity tended to be lower for lymphocytes from rats fed high-fat diets than for those fed low-fat diets, irrespective of the principal saturated fatty acid present. (Natural killer or NK cells, which are a subpopulation of lymphocytes, attack appropriate tumor or toxic cells.)

In another experiment to determine the immuno-modulatory effects of specific dietary fatty acids, weanling male rats were fed high-fat diets that differed according to the principal fatty acids present (Wanten and Calder 2007). The nine diets used differed in their contents of palmitic (C16), oleic (C18:1), linoleic (C18:2, omega-6), and alpha-linolenic acids (C18:3 omega-3). Predictably, the fat composition of the diet significantly influenced the fatty acid composition of the serum and of spleen lymphocytes. The proliferation of lymphocytes and NK cells decreased as the level of monounsaturated acid (C18:1, omega-9, as in olive oil) in the diet increased.

NK cell activity increased as the *saturated* palmitic acid content of the diet increased. Surprise! The inference is that saturated fats containing palmitic acid are healthier than monounsaturated fats when it comes to our immune system. Perhaps this is why human milk fat ranges from a 20 to 25% palmitic acid content.

Collective evidence suggests that the condition of protein malnutrition also contributes to abnormal levels of inflammation. The primary goal of nutritional support in inflammatory disease is to provide adequate energy and protein to meet the body's requirements for tissue repair and restored cellular function, thus protecting us from infection.

An effect of modulation of inflammatory and immune parameters has been studied in patients with rheumatic and inflammatory disease receiving dietary supplementation of omega-3 (fish oils, spinach, nuts, flax seed, etc.). Investigators in Europe, the

United States, and Australia described consistent improvement in tender joints of rheumatoid arthritis with omega-3 supplementation. Improvements in morning stiffness were also reported. Some patients with rheumatoid arthritis are able to discontinue nonsteroidal anti-inflammatory drugs (NSAIDs) while receiving omega-3 fatty acids (Goldberg and Katz 2007).

Given the poor prognosis and high cost of care for surgical patients with acute inflammatory responses, immunomodulation of this hyperresponse represents an important priority for research in nutritional medicine. In the research this book focuses upon, this goal has been pursued—with significant success—through use of special lipids. Manipulation of macrophage by use of omega-3 polyunsaturated fatty acids may reduce this cellular immune response, thereby reducing inflammation. As more data are obtained on the use of special lipids, possibly a new generation of diets based on saturated fats such as monolaurin/extra virgin coconut oil/palm kernel oil rather than omega-6 fats (which are pro-inflammatory) could be developed to better support immune function and reduce inflammation.

As a pertinent example, intravenous lipid solutions as parts of Total Parenteral Nutrition (TPN) are now standard in most hospital centers. TPN is normally used following surgery, when feeding by mouth or using the gut is not possible. TPN is given when a person's digestive system cannot absorb nutrients due to chronic disease or, alternatively, if a person's nutrient requirement cannot be met by enteral feeding (tube feeding). Until recently, the most common and frequently used lipid formula contained predominantly long-chain triglycerides of the omega-6 series. Controversy and concern presently exist about the immunosuppressive effects of this fat source, as repeatedly noted in our discussion. These concerns are mainly based on laboratory data, as clinical studies are sparse. Some investigators, however, have pointed out that long-chain polyunsaturated triglyceride lipid emulsions impair macrophage functions. To avoid this problem, lipid emulsions now usually contain 50% medium-chain saturated triglycerides and 50% long-chain triglycerides. These newer formulas produce less deleterious effects on immune response than the traditional lipid source.

The saturated alkylglycerol ethers (similar but not identical to saturated glycerol) from shark liver have been used for more than fifty years as a natural supplement. Numerous articles suggest that alkylglycerols have been used successfully in the treatment of neoplastic disorders (cancer) and as an immune booster in infectious diseases.

Proposed mechanisms of action suggest various possibilities, including induction of apoptosis (cell suicide) of neoplastic cells, suppression of cell-cell communication, inhibition of angiogenesis (developing new blood vessels), and promotion of the efflux of cytotoxic chemotherapeutic agents.

Preliminary data suggest that alkylglycerol (which is an ether form) and monolaurin (an ester form of lauric acid) have similar pharmacological effects. While this information is highly suggestive, specific clinical experiments are needed to confirm these laboratory findings.

Fat Effects on Autoimmune Disease

An autoimmune disease is a condition caused by the reaction of antibodies to substances occurring naturally in the body. It has been found that diets with qualitative and quantitative differences in fat content have a profound influence on the manifestation and progression of the autoimmune syndrome.

Lupus Erythematosus

Systemic lupus erythematosus (SLE) is a chronic, inflammatory autoimmune disorder. It may affect the skin, joints, kidneys, and other organs.

Normally, the immune system controls the body's defenses against infection. In SLE and other autoimmune diseases, these defenses are turned against oneself (the body organs) as rogue immune cells attack tissues. Antibodies may be produced that can react against the body's blood cells, organs, and tissues. These lead immune cells to attack the affected systems, producing a chronic (long-term) disease. The mechanism or cause of autoimmune diseases is not fully known, but many researchers suspect that it occurs following infection with an organism that looks similar to particular proteins in the body, which are later mistaken for the organism and wrongly targeted for attack. The disease affects nine times as many women as men. It may occur at any age but appears most often in people between the ages of 10 and 50 years.

The influence of dietary fat on autoimmunity in lupus-prone mice was studied in order to elucidate the effects of dietary lipids on the immune system. (A full discussion can be found in the article

"Modulatory Effects of Dietary Lipids on Immune System Functions," *Immunology and Cell Biology,* Vol. 78, pp. 31–39, 2000.) Female weanling mice (because 80–90% of human cases are female) were presented four diets differing in quantity and type of fat. Their immunologic response was then studied by a variety of tests at 4 and 7 months of age. Few differences were seen among the four groups at 4 months of age. At 7 months mice receiving diets high in unsaturated fat demonstrated hyper-responsiveness (a negative reaction since it indicates autoimmunity) to injected sheep red blood cells. These results indicate that diets high in fat, particularly unsaturated fat, influence immune responses. A prudent fat diet (no one fat in excess) can reduce the development of disease by maintaining normal immune responses.

Crohn's Disease

Crohn's Disease is an Inflammatory Bowel Disease (IBD) and auto-immune condition of the small intestine. Many suggest that Crohn's Disease is an advanced case of Irritable Bowel Syndrome that has progressed to this inflammatory and immune-related stage.

Gut-associated lymphoid tissue is the major inductive site of the mucosal immune system, which is functionally independent of the systemic immune system. Again, it is worth repeating that both the amount and type of dietary fat modulate intestinal immune function. In particular, unsaturated fatty acids at high concentrations have a greater suppressive effect on cell-mediated immunity than do saturated fats. Fat absorption by the intestinal mucosa increases release of cytokine (a messenger molecule that is secreted by a cell) from intestinal epithelial cells. In Crohn's disease, intravenous nutrition often induces remission, possibly by reducing antigenic load on activated immune cells in the intestine. Taking supplemental dietary fish oil or flax seed oil apparently tends to prevent relapse of Crohn's disease. Because dietary fat intake is closely associated with immunological function of the intestinal mucosa, careful manipulation of dietary fat should be considered in the management of this disease. Medium-chain (C8-C12) saturated triglycerides (MCTs) or C12 monoglyceride like monolaurin should be considered healthier fats when compared to highly unsaturated fats.

CHAPTER 8

The Role of Fats in Cancer

In recent decades, the incidence of cancer has increased in industrial societies. This may be explained, at least in part, by longer life expectancy and the fact that cancer occurs more frequently with increasing age. The question has been raised as to whether the amount and type of fat consumed influences the occurrence and growth of malignant cells. In particular, the trans fatty acids, which are so prevalent in margarines and other foods, have been scrutinized. I've always claimed that butter is better than margarines containing trans fats. Nevertheless, increased fat intake does contribute to more frequent occurrence of cancer. The amount and kind of fat influence tumorigenesis (tumor formation). However, the touting of polyunsaturated fatty acids by the American Heart Association presents special problems to individuals genetically predisposed to cancer. High amounts of fats and especially polyunsaturated fatty acids stimulate the action of carcinogens (cancer-causing agents) that are introduced into the modern diet. This question of fat in our diet and its role in initiating or supporting tumorigenesis is addressed in this chapter.

Much of what was written in a previous chapter about fats and the immune system is applicable to cancer formation since our immune system is what saves us from cells prone to uncontrolled growth.

High-Fat Diets and Cancer

Tannenbaum and his associates reported in 1942 an increased incidence of tumors in rats fed high-fat diets (Tannenbaum 1942). This led to a great deal of experimental work on the effect of high fat intake on cancers. In addition, epidemiology data suggested a correlation between high fat intake and increased incidence of tumors consistently observed, particularly breast, colon, and pancreatic cancers. In other organs, such as the lung, fat consumption appears to have less effect on cancer appearance.

Detailed accounts on the subject can be found in *Dietary Fats and Health,* edited by E.G. Perkins and W.J. Visek (1983). As described by K.K. Carroll and co-workers in one of the book's chapters, both the epidemiological and experimental data suggest that fat in general, and unsaturated vegetable oils in particular, lead to more frequent occurrence of mammary cancers. Colon tumors especially occur more frequently in populations on high fat-intake diets.

Considerable thought has been given to the question of whether the high caloric content or the structure of fats is responsible for their tumorigenic effect. ("Tumorigenic" refers to an agent that may initiate or promote the growth of tumors.) In this same book, Kritchevsky and co-workers demonstrated that high caloric intake itself favors tumorigenesis. Most lipid researchers were inclined to accept this theory. However, it is hard to deny the greater effects of specific fats. Many experiments have been carried out regarding the action of specific fats on the effect of various cancer-causing chemicals. A number of the reports are summarized in the American Oil Chemists' Society's monographs *The Pharmacological Effects of Lipids,* Volumes I–III.

Polyunsaturated Fatty Acids and Cancer

There is unanimous agreement that fats in general and polyunsaturated vegetable oils in particular favor the development of tumors. So why does the American Heart Association (AHA) keep telling us to eat more polyunsaturated fatty acids? (The full answer to this question is found in Chapter 9; in short, it has to do with old consensus thinking about atherosclerosis and what I call "the Cholesterol-Heart Hypothesis.") The AHA has only focused on the effect of polyunsaturated fatty acids on cholesterol levels; other deleterious factors are ignored (again, see Chapter 9). In fact, the feeding of unsaturated vegetable oil enhanced the number, size, and speed of appearance of mammary and colon tumors in lab experiments. Present laboratory results on the relationship of polyunsaturated fats and cancer agree with human epidemiological experiences.

The metabolic mechanisms by which particular unsaturated vegetable oils act have been variously explained. In reviewing the subject, especially from the standpoint of mammary cancer, K.K. Carroll suggested that adverse effects on the DNA repair system, on immuno-competence, and on membrane structure were the reasons that polyunsaturated fatty acids help promote cancer (see Chapter 14 of *The Pharmacological Effect of Lipids,* Vol. III).

It is now well accepted that unsaturated fats increase the permeability and fluidity of cell membranes. As a result, the sensitivity or permeability of cell membranes to carcinogens may be increased by consumption of unsaturated fats. Although not all answers are clear-cut, it seems apparent that the consumption of large amounts of polyunsaturated vegetable oils is not in the public interest. What constitutes a healthy diet in regard to fat intake seems to be championed by two different groups with quite incompatible conclusions. It has not been proven by the American Heart Association that increased consumption of polyunsaturated fatty acids can prevent atherosclerosis. Meanwhile we hear from the American Cancer Society that there are certain risks associated with the ingestion of polyunsaturated fats. Is our choice therefore one of dying from heart disease (low polyunsaturated fat intake) or cancer (high intake)? **The answer seems to be that moderation and variation in fat intake is the best recommendation.**

Studies also show a relationship between increased amounts of certain dietary polyunsaturates and *amyloidosis* (a condition marked by the accumulation of a protein-based substance called amyloid in the body's organs). This may lead to liver disease, intestinal damage and obstruction, gonadal damage, or hypertension. Increased intake of polyunsaturated fats leads to increased lipid peroxides. These oxygenated unsaturated bonds (peroxides) can lead to an increase in either atherosclerosis or cancer.

Olive oil, which is rich in monounsaturated oleic acid ($C18:1$, omega-9) and saturated fats, does not exert tumor-promoting effects as strongly as vegetable omega-6 polyunsaturated fats. More recently, it has been demonstrated that the omega-3 polyunsaturated fatty acids derived from fish and marine mammals lack tumor-promoting effects (as compared to the vegetable oils). **Therefore, a "good" or "bad" effect of polyunsaturated fat depends on the amount and specific kind of fat in the diet.**

It seems appropriate to warn people about eating foods that are fried or overheated in polyunsaturated oils. Foods prepared in commercial establishments are particularly suspect, since these polyunsaturated fats (oils) are heated repeatedly, resulting in the greater formation of dangerous lipid peroxides. Small amounts of such heated polyunsaturates (peroxides) form polymerized (varnish-like) toxic chemicals, which can cause tissue damage and even death. It is likely that most, if not all, of the carcinogenicity is due to the breakdown products (lipid peroxides) of unsaturated fats, especially when they are overheated repeatedly. Some of the potentially carcinogenic lipid peroxides are extremely toxic; they can be formed easily from polyunsaturated fats by autoxidation, the result of heat and air oxygen. Heating polyunsaturated fats can also produce polycyclic and aromatic hydrocarbons, additional toxic and potentially carcinogenic substances. So much for the health "benefits" of using polyunsaturated fats for cooking or frying. Tropical oils (coconut oil and palm kernel oil), on the other hand, are highly saturated and do not form these harmful peroxides. Despite their favorable stability, these oils were irrationally removed from movie theaters for popping corn and replaced, thanks to the soybean lobby, by the more oxidizable and dangerous polyunsaturated vegetable oils. Butter and lard (saturated fats) are also preferred over polyunsaturated oils for cooking at higher temperatures.

Politics/money not science seems to control what we are told is healthy.

Medium-Chain Triglycerides and Cancer

Since about 1975, increasing attention has been devoted to the importance of the *type* (fatty acid profile) as well as the *amount* of dietary fat in experimental mammary, colon, and pancreatic tumorigenesis. Saturated fatty acids (C12:0 and shorter) are generally reported to have less effect on tumor development than long-chain polyunsaturated fatty acids. Coconut oil, which contains ~50% lauric acid (C12:0), does not promote mammary tumorigenesis. Babayan and co-workers (1989) have studied medium-chain triglycerides (MCT) over the past five decades. MCT is a semi-synthetic oil derived from coconut oil. MCT oils, however, contain more C8:0 and C10:0 fatty acids than C12:0, as compared to coconut oil. Based on these studies, it is now known that medium-chain triglyceride oils are unique among fats.

MCTs are utilized by the body more like simple carbohydrates than conventional long-chain fatty acid (LCFA) triglycerides. For example, MCTs are rapidly absorbed and transported directly to the liver via the portal vein rather than via the lymphatic system, as are longer-chain triglycerides. Moreover, due to their greater water solubility and smaller size, MCTs are transported through the circulation bound to albumin rather than being incorporated into globules (chylomicrons), as are long-chain triglycerides. Again, in contrast to LC fats, MCTs are rapidly oxidized for energy in the mitochondria of the liver and other tissues and are not stored in fat deposits, nor incorporated into cell membranes to any great extent.

These unique characteristics of MCTs suggest that they would be prime candidates as dietary fats, since they do not promote cancer and have a lower caloric value (8.3/gram instead of 9.0) than other fats. While chemically defined as fats in a biochemical sense, the MCTs behave energetically more like simple carbohydrates. Currently MCTs are being promoted for sport bars since they provide energy equivalent of carbohydrates without the necessary production of insulin.

Effects of Fats and Calories on Carcinogenesis

We do not understand the mechanism by which carcinogenesis is enhanced by dietary fat. We know that a minimum level of essential fatty acids (EFAs) is necessary for mammary tumor development, and that this level probably exceeds the normal requirement (approximately 3%) for dietary intake. Once the minimum levels of EFAs have been supplied, the calorie contribution of the dietary fat may account for its enhancement of carcinogenesis. In this regard, we must recognize that the efficiency with which dietary energy is utilized is known to increase as the fat content of the diet is raised. Hence, high-fat diets will provide more net energy than low-fat diets with the same total caloric value. Modulation of host fat and calorie intake has been previously proposed as affecting immunity.

Diets rich in omega-6 polyunsaturated fatty acids are significantly

TABLE 8.1

Percent by weight of total fatty acids

Oil or Fat	Unsat./ Sat. Ratio	Saturated		
		Capric Acid C10:0	Lauric Acid C12:0	Myristic Acid C14:0
Almond oil	9.7	-	-	-
Beef Tallow	0.9	-	-	3
Butterfat (cow)	0.5	3	3	11
Butterfat (goat)	0.5	7	3	9
Butterfat (human)	1.0	2	5	8
Canola Oil	15.7	-	-	-
Cocoa Butter	0.6	-	-	-
Cod Liver Oil	2.9	-	-	8
Coconut Oil	0.1	6	47	18
Corn Oil (Maize Oil)	6.7	-	-	-
Cottonseed Oil	2.8	-	-	1
Flaxseed Oil	9.0	-	-	-
Grape seed Oil	7.3	-	-	-
Lard (Pork fat)	1.2	-	-	2
Olive Oil	4.6	-	-	-
Palm Oil	1.0	-	-	1
Palm Olein	1.3	-	-	1
Palm Kernel Oil	0.2	4	48	16
Peanut Oil	4.0	-	-	-
Safflower Oil*	10.1	-	-	-
Sesame Oil	6.6	-	-	-
Soybean Oil	5.7	-	-	-
Sunflower Oil*	7.3	-	-	-

Saturated		Mono unsaturated	Poly unsaturated	
Palmitic Acid C16:0	Stearic Acid C18:0	Oleic Acid C18:1	Linoleic Acid (ω6) C18:2	Alpha Linolenic Acid (ω3) C18:3
7	2	69	17	-
24	19	43	3	1
27	12	29	2	1
25	12	27	3	1
25	8	35	9	1
4	2	62	22	10
25	38	32	3	-
17	-	22	5	-
9	3	6	2	-
11	2	28	58	1
22	3	19	54	1
3	7	21	16	53
8	4	15	73	-
26	14	44	10	-
13	3	71	10	1
45	4	40	10	-
37	4	46	11	-
8	3	15	2	-
11	2	48	32	-
7	2	13	78	-
9	4	41	45	-
11	4	24	54	7
7	5	19	68	1

immunosuppressive. Mice were fed diets enriched with linoleic (POLY, omega-6), oleic (MONO, omega-9), palmitic (SAT), or eicosapentaenoic (FISH, omega-3) fatty acids. Several weeks later, these mice were injected with methylcholanthrene, a carcinogen. Immune studies were performed several months afterward. The mice fed the POLY diet survived poorly, and many were infected with *Mycoplasma pulmonis*. They were the only mice to experience significant immunosuppression. Aspirin partially reversed the immunosuppression of this POLY diet, which possibly provides us with another reason to take aspirin. Mice fed the FISH omega-3 diet were not immunosuppressed. It was tentatively concluded that diets rich in omega-6 polyunsaturated fats but not omega-3 polyunsaturated fats predispose animals to suppression of certain mediated immune responses that can be "triggered" by infection and/or exposure to carcinogens.

Because of high levels of dietary vegetable oil intake, excessive omega-6 polyunsaturated fatty acid metabolites can encourage infection via prolonged inflammation and immunosuppression. Vegetarians take note. Lipids can influence host immunity by altering membrane structure and metabolic function. This being the case, additional investigations are essential to answer questions regarding the present levels and properties of various essential fatty acids used in hospital total parenteral nutrition (TPN) lipid emulsions. Combining omega-3 polyunsaturated fatty acid (fish oil) and monolaurin into a synthetic lipid TPN emulsion may decrease infection and improve survival rates by producing fewer inflammatory fatty acids. **The inclusion of omega-3 polyunsaturated fatty acids and monolaurin in TPN emulsions, as well as normal diets, may**

provide important benefits in the prevention of disease and enhancement of health.

Tumor necrosis factor (TNF) is a macrophage-derived peptide (a small protein) that has anti-tumor action and modulates immune and inflammatory reactions. Dietary fatty acids can modulate TNF production. Dietary omega-3 polyunsaturated fatty acids enhance TNF production and secretion. Macrophages from mice fed the high omega-3 diet produced an eightfold increase in the TNF compared to mice fed omega-6 diets (Hardardóttir and Kinsella 1992).

The drug indomethacin (which works by inhibiting the production of prostaglandins, molecules known to increase inflammation) caused an increase in the TNF production by macrophages from mice on all diets, but macrophages from mice on the high omega-3 diet produced 70% more TNF than macrophages from mice on the other diets. These results explain why consumption of omega-3 polyunsaturated fatty acids enhances TNF production by macrophages. **Omega-3 fatty acids help reduce the production of inflammatory prostaglandins.**

Given the above information, it is reasonable to limit rather than increase the amount of omega-6 polyunsaturated fatty acid intake in human diets, since omega-6 fatty acids produce inflammatory prostaglandins. In addition, the amount of vitamin E and other metabolites necessary to prevent lipid peroxidation of polyunsaturated fatty acids should be considered.

A prudent diet would include medium-chain fats (coconut and palm kernel oils), monounsaturated C18:1 (omega-9) fats, and omega-3 fats, while limiting the amount of long-chain saturated, trans, and omega-6 unsaturated fats. A balanced healthy diet would include modest amounts of fats, proteins, and carbohydrates. Rather than a specific dietary nutrient, ill health is more likely caused by overeating and a sedentary lifestyle, particularly when accompanied by stress. My personal experiences suggest that the saturated lipid supplement Lauricidin should become a significant part of a daily healthy diet.

Cholesterol and Cancer

While not a fat, cholesterol is a lipid, and its effects in cancer formation are significant. Since a great deal of attention on cholesterol relates to heart disease, its role in cancer is unfortunately often ignored. The immune system in men with hypo/hypercholesterolemia is different. A considerable volume of epidemiological evidence indicates that relative hypocholesterolemia (low cholesterol levels: <160 mg/dl) in apparently healthy individuals is associated with increased mortality from cancer and other non-atherosclerotic causes of death. Of particular note is the fact that patients with AIDS and cancer frequently have low cholesterol values.

A study was conducted to better understand the reasons for these unexplained associations and their underlying effects (Muldoon et al. 1997). Nineteen healthy adult men with a mean age of 46 years and a mean total cholesterol concentration of 151 mg/ml constituted a low-cholesterol group. They were compared with 39 men of a similar age but whose total cholesterol averaged 261 mg/ml. Relative to the high-cholesterol group, hypocholesterolemic men had significantly fewer circulating lymphocytes, fewer total T cells, and fewer CD8+ cells. In addition to these studies, research with 121 healthy women indicated that their low cholesterol values were inversely associated with characteristic measures of depression and anxiety (Suarez 1999). These data provide evidence of differences in healthy individuals with hypo- and hypercholesterolemia. Either is a risk factor but not a cause of ill health.

Reflecting on my early (1972) finding that hypocholesterolemic drugs like clofibrate shorten the life span of tumor-bearing animals, it seems prudent *not* to lower cholesterol levels too far. After I experienced a heart attack in Germany in 1980, it was recommended that I take the (then-current) drug of choice, clofibrate, which I obviously refused. "Why won't you follow our recommendation?" asked the attending physician. I replied that my research indicated that clofibrate shortens the lives of tumor-bearing animals. "Those are only animal studies" was his arrogant rebuttal. Less than a year later clofibrate was taken off the market because it was associated with increased numbers of cancer reports.

People who have especially low levels of total cholesterol have higher rather than lower risk of disease. The relationship between cholesterol and cancer is actually a protective one for cholesterol. Every cell in the body is provided with a cell membrane or "raincoat" that keeps it from being dissolved in the watery fluids of the bloodstream. Cholesterol is a vital substance. Cholesterol is the precursor of every sex and steroid hormone in the body. **The body needs this important lipid and uses numerous substances to guarantee its formation. Cholesterol can be made from fatty acids, amino acids, or even glucose. No other chemical in our body has so many options for its formation.**

A 17-year study at the University of Basel in Switzerland found that men with the lowest levels of cholesterol (less than 199 mg/ml) have a 70% greater risk of stomach cancer after age 60. They have a 100% greater risk of lung cancer, and a 307% greater risk of colon cancer (Eichholzer et al. 2000). Even when the scientists introduced control factors for smoking and consumption of beta-carotene, vitamin C, and vitamin E, men with cholesterol below 199 mg/dl had a 770% greater risk of prostate cancer by age 60.

It has been frustrating for me to deal with the common but now known to be false notion that cholesterol is bad. This perception is fostered by the greed of drug and food companies who sell anti-cholesterol drugs and cholesterol/fat-free foods. It is deceitful marketing rather than good science when contrary opinions, as found in this book, are not even considered.

As you will read in the next chapter on atherosclerosis, cholesterol is part of a protective mechanism and not the cause of heart disease. Its high association with heart disease can be explained by its presence to help protect blood vessels under an unspecified attack.

Monoglycerides of Bitter Melon

The use of herbs to treat illness has its roots in an ancient holistic healing tradition that originated in Asia more than three thousand years ago. Largely discounted by 19th- and 20th-century practitioners of Western medicine, healing practices incorporating herbal remedies from traditional Chinese medicine, Japanese Kampo, and Indian Ayurveda are gaining acceptance in the West as we enter the 21st century. One such plant extract, bitter melon, has gained recent attention. It was exciting to read about the historical role of bitter melon in curing cancer and other medical conditions. These remarkable studies reveal a possible association between bitter melon and Lauricidin, and they help us discern the biochemical mechanisms influenced by the medium-chain monoglycerides like monolaurin. This information gives us clues to new uses for a pure and accessible form of the healthiest fatty acid, lauric acid in the form of monolaurin. We are only beginning to understand the many nutriceutical benefits of various foods.

Bitter melon *(Momordica charantia)* is a plant that grows in tropical areas of Asia, the Caribbean, and South America, and it has a long history of use as a traditional medicine. It has been reported that bitter melon has antidiabetic, antiviral, antioxidative, and antineoplastic (anti-cancer) effects (Basch et al. 2003). An identified fraction of the seeds and fruits of bitter melon has therapeutic effects by acting as an inhibitor of P-glycoprotein (P-gp). P-gp belongs to a family of proteins that transport material from cells. P-gp protein acts as an energy-dependent drug efflux pump. This means that it prevents cellular accumulation of a broad range of cytotoxic drugs by withdrawing the drug from the cell.

It has been acknowledged that the over-expression of P-glycoprotein on the surface of cells, particularly tumor cells, causes multidrug resistance. Modulators of P-gp function can therefore restore the sensitivity of resistant cells to drugs. Such modulators may increase the effective use of more chemotherapeutic drugs, especially those drugs formerly thought to be totally useless. To isolate the P-gp inhibitory substance(s) in bitter melon, various concentrations of methanol were used by T. Konishi et al. (2004) to determine which concentration would be most effective for extracting the active substance. The fraction having the most P-gp inhibiting activity was finally analyzed and identified to be sn1-monopalmitin. Other monoglycerides with a variety of hydrocarbon-chain length were tested and also found be inhibitory toward P-gp. These data suggest that one active effect of bitter melon could therefore be due to the monoglycerides and other inhibitory lipoproteins containing monoglycerides. Working with pure monoglycerides—including sn1-monolaurin (Lauricidin, C12), sn1-monomyristin (C14), and sn1-monopalmitin (C16)—revealed that all have similar activity. In separate studies of my own as well as research by others, only the C12 monoglyceride (monolaurin, a.k.a. Lauricidin) has been shown to have high antibacterial and antiviral properties.

It is surprising that simple monoglycerides (C8-C16) in bitter melon were found to be P-gp-inhibiting substances. Although a variety of functions for monoglycerides has been reported (Boyle & German 1996; Emilio 2003), the modulation of P-gp functions by monoglycerides had not been previously reported. This may be a newly discovered function for monoglycerides. One could conclude that one of the physiological roles for sn1-monoglycerides is reflected in its modulation of P-gp functions.

It is important to emphasize that the sn2-monoglyceride produced from oral dietary triglycerides (fats) by specific esterases in the small intestine *is not an important active monoglyceride*. This is because the sn2-monoglyceride (although active topically) is readily absorbed and quickly converted into the inactive triglyceride. Therefore, it is only when natural or synthetic sn1-monoglycerides like monolaurin are taken orally that they have any significant biological activity.

Bitter melon extracts have also proven to be good antibiotics. Both bitter melon and monolaurin have been documented with *in vitro* antiviral activity against numerous viruses including Epstein-Barr, herpes, and HIV. In an *in vivo* study, a leaf extract of bitter melon demonstrated the ability to increase resistance to viral infections, as well as to provide an immunostimulant effect in humans and animals. This takes place by increasing natural killer cell activity as well as the production of *interferon* (a complex glycoprotein produced by cells in response to a virus or bacterium that inhibits virus development). Thus, bitter melon and monolaurin have many similar biochemical properties.

CHAPTER 9

Atherosclerosis and Infection

If you know the following, you need not read this chapter:

- Cholesterol is not a deadly poison, but a substance vital to most living cells.
- Your body produces two-thirds of the cholesterol you need. This production *increases* when you eat only small amounts of cholesterol and *decreases* when you eat large amounts.
- Many of the cholesterol-lowering drugs are dangerous to your health and *may even shorten your life.*
- Cholesterol-lowering drugs *may* only lower heart-disease morbidity but not total mortality. These drugs have other undesirable effects (potential for cancer, depression, suicide, muscle problems, etc.).
- People whose blood cholesterol is low develop just as many plaques in their blood vessels as people whose cholesterol is high.
- People with atherosclerosis live longer than people with low cholesterol.

Many of the facts in this chapter have been presented in scientific journals and books for decades, but proponents of the Cholesterol-Heart Hypothesis never tell them to the public. Why? Unfortunately, the reason is money. The Cholesterol-Heart Hypothesis and the whole cholesterol phobia campaign have created immense prosperity for researchers, doctors, drug producers, and the food industry. In fact, cholesterol is NOT a cause of heart disease but rather a protective mechanism of the body to heal vessel injury.

Atherosclerosis is the principal cause of coronary artery disease (CAD) and is the single largest killer of both men and women in the United States. The word "atherosclerosis" is of Greek origin and literally means "gruel hardening." The focal accumulation of lipids and the thickening of arterial walls identify it. CAD refers to the presence of atherosclerotic changes within the walls of the coronary arteries, which cause impairment or obstruction of normal blood flow, resulting in an inadequate supply of blood to myocardial (heart) tissue. CAD is a progressive disease process that generally begins in childhood and manifests clinically in mid to late adulthood. The distribution of lipid and connective tissue in the atherosclerotic lesion determines whether the blood vessel is stable or at risk of rupture, thrombosis, and further problems.

Approximately 14 million Americans have CAD. Each year, 1.5 million individuals develop acute myocardial infarction (a.k.a. heart attack, the most deadly presentation of CAD), and 500,000 of these individuals die. Heart attack survivors continue to have a poor prognosis, and their risk of mortality and morbidity is 1.5–15 times greater than that of the rest of the population. This fact remains true despite a 30% reduction in mortality and morbidity from CAD over the past three decades (statistics from the American Heart Association). Many factors have led to this decrease, including the introduction of coronary care units, bypass surgery (e.g. coronary artery bypass graft), thrombolytic therapy, angioplasty, and a tremendous emphasis on lifestyle modification.

Three Theories of Atherosclerosis Genesis

The Encrustation Theory

This theory, proposed by Karl Freiherr von Rokitansky in 1851, suggested that atherosclerosis begins in the intima (the innermost lining of a blood vessel) with deposition of thrombus (blood clot) and its subsequent organization by the infiltration of fibroblasts and *secondary lipid deposition.*

The Lipid Theory

In 1856, German pathologist Rudolf Virchow proposed that atherosclerosis starts with lipid infiltration into the arterial wall and its interaction with cellular and extracellular elements, causing "intimal proliferation." Wladimir Sergius von Ignatowsky in 1908 fed animal foods to rabbits. He attributed the production of atherosclerosis to protein intoxication. A Russian, Nikolai Nikolajewitsch Anitschkow, in 1913 carried out similar experiments and attributed the lesions to dietary cholesterol. Anitschkow's lipid theory, now popular, should never have been accepted since rabbits are vegetarians and normally not exposed to dietary cholesterol intake. His theory is what has come to be called the Cholesterol-

Heart Hypothesis. As the backbone of the whole cholesterol-phobia campaign, this theory has continued to be championed decades later for monetary gain even when good modern science contradicts its old tenets. Ongoing acceptance of the Cholesterol-Heart Hypothesis continues to bring income to the segment of the medical industry that evolved around it, yet few studies show the benefits of cholesterol lowering on overall mortality statistics.

The Theory of Response to Endothelial Injury

In 1858, the insightful Rudolf Virchow wrote a book titled *Cellular Pathology* in which he formulated his concept (stated above) that changes in cells account for diseases in organs. Subsequently, Virchow postulated the response-to-injury model of atherosclerosis. Modern research and new knowledge of vascular injury continue to punch holes in the Cholesterol-Heart Hypothesis. Today Virchow's earlier concept of atherosclerosis (response to injury) appears more viable.

Virchow described mural thrombosis (inflammatory damage to arterial intima). This damage increases intimal permeability to plasma products like cholesterol, degeneration of arterial wall, deposition of plasma lipids in plaques, and finally fibrosis and calcification of plaques. Currently, a re-emerging theory on the role of inflammation and infection in atherosclerosis seems to better explain many clinical facts not considered by other theories.

The response-to-injury hypothesis renewed by Russell Ross in 1993 provides more insight into the complex mechanisms whereby hyperlipidemia perpetuates progressive atherosclerosis. **Physical,**

chemical, or bacterial/viral injury to the lining of arteries sets off a process, which is probably an attempt by cholesterol at healing the injury but which leads instead to atherosclerosis. It has also been found that chemical agents such as homocysteine can produce a similar series of events leading to atherosclerosis. Any injury of connective tissue can lead to adherence of platelets followed by release of factors that stimulate intimal smooth muscle proliferation. Current studies indicate that the effects of chronic hyperlipidemia are complex. The increase in serum cholesterol may be an attempt by the body to heal a previous injury, and not be a cause of the injury.

From an evolutionary point of view, cholesterol is the most sophisticated molecule in our biological world. In the primordial origin of animate things, cholesterol was not found in lower forms of life such as bacteria. It was only when oxygen became available that cholesterol appeared in nature. In chemical evolution, this molecule with its highly developed structure was and is necessary for insects and fungi to exist and grow. In other words, cholesterol is an essential component of more complex living things. All cells in higher biological forms have the ability to make cholesterol. From a teleological argument of evolution (seeking the ultimate purpose of a design or function), biological systems would not make or require a substance that would be toxic or harmful to it.

All evolutionary changes occur for a definite protective purpose or to gain a biological advantage. Cholesterol is the most highly developed chemical in nature. Cholesterol is the precursor of many substances essential to life such as bile acids, sex hormones, and vitamin D. Cholesterol is part of every cell in the human body.

The brain contains the highest concentration of this "deadly" sterol. Cholesterol is one of the few if not the only substance in our body that can use amino acids, carbohydrates, or fatty acids for its formation. Because of these various remarkable metabolic schemes, cholesterol can hardly be called a culprit in the epidemic of poor human health.

The frequent clinical observations that most, but not all, people with heart disease have high cholesterol values seem to support the "cholesterol theory" of heart disease. The conundrum of "causation" versus "correlation" is an age-old medical question and an important one when it comes to understanding cardiovascular disease. Think about a child who has seen a number of house fires.

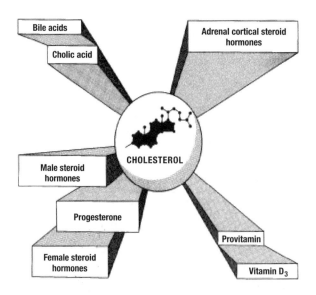

Figure 9.1: SOME DERIVATIVES OF CHOLESTEROL
Courtesy of G.J. Brisson, PhD.

He/she observes that firemen are always present at house fires and concludes that firemen must cause these fires. The child does not yet understand that the firemen are actually there to save the day. It's the same thing with the Cholesterol-Heart Hypothesis, where cholesterol is seen as an evil cause of cardiovascular disease simply because it is *highly associated* with the disease. A conclusion that cholesterol is elevated as a protective mechanism—not a cause of cardiovascular disease—is not even considered by those promoting the "cholesterol theory" of heart disease.

A similar example of faulty cause-effect arguments is the observation that high glucose is a cause of diabetes. Lowering sugar in our diet or even using insulin does not cure diabetes. High sugar is associated with but not the cause of diabetes. Likewise, we are focusing on the wrong question when we ask, "How do we reduce cholesterol values?" The pathetic truth of the matter is that the promotion of low-cholesterol and low-fat diets and/or the use of drugs for "better health" is aggressively supported by the greed of the food and drug industry and not by good science.

An eight-year study that was completed in 2006 involving nearly 49,000 women 50–79 years of age concluded the following: There was no difference in heart attack and stroke incidence between those assigned to a low-fat diet and those who ate whatever they pleased (Howard et al. 2006).

Making good dietary choices does really matter, but it is the types of fat, not necessarily the amount, that is most important. However, keep in mind that too many calories from both fat and carbohydrates will lead to weight gain, which will increase risks of breast cancer, colon cancer, and heart disease. Although not mentioned in the study, low-fat foods are generally higher in salt and carbohydrate content, both of which should be included in moderation for a healthy diet.

Cholesterol and Statins

For almost a century, cholesterol has been implicated as a cause of heart disease because of its association with it. During all this time, efforts to reduce heart disease by lowering cholesterol have failed. Support for the idea that cholesterol is not the cause of heart disease came from observations of Dr. Hans Kaunitz, a pathologist from Columbia University. The interested reader is encouraged to read his many papers, which can be found online.

Dr. Kaunitz and I became good friends after meeting in the early 1960s at an American Oil Chemists' Society meeting. We shared the same idea that the cholesterol accumulation in vascular vessels is a protective mechanism rather than a cause of plaque formation. Where there is injury to the endothelial tissue by chemicals, microorganisms, etc., the body produces more cholesterol to protect the site of injury.

Because of the current popularity of the Cholesterol-Heart Hypothesis, efforts have been solely directed to reduce cholesterol by diet or drugs. Today the most important drugs are hydroxymethylglutaryl coenzymeA (HMG-CoA) reductase inhibitors, known collectively as "statins." These statin inhibitors block the rate-limiting enzyme in cholesterol synthesis. These drugs act by inhibiting the formulation of isoprene units which are used to form cholesterol. However, other important nonsterol compounds, such as coenzyme Q10 (CoQ10), are also derived from the same synthetic pathway. CoQ10 is an essential carrier in the mitochondrial respiratory chain that participates in cell and heart oxidative activities. Simvastatin and other HMG-CoA reductase inhibitors have been documented to lower serum concentrations of CoQ10. It has been suggested that the adverse effects of myopathy caused by HMG-CoA reductase inhibitors are due to CoQ10 deficiency in the tissue mitochondria, especially heart muscle.

It is important to point out that cholesterol needs **six isoprene units** for its formation. This same pathway is also used to make coenzyme Q10. Coenzyme Q10 needs **ten isoprene units,** thus its formation is more adversely affected than cholesterol production by the statin drugs. Even your doctor is not aware of this potential problem.

A decrease in tissue coenzyme Q10 will have adverse effects on both skeletal muscle and myocardial function. It has been shown that skeletal muscle pathology such as myalgia and rhabdomyolysis can be a consequence of statin therapy (Tomlinson and Mangione 2005). This effect is particularly noticeable in the elderly, which is the major population using this drug. Interference with the mitochondrial energy production is part of the toxicity of this class of drugs, and it is becoming increasingly more evident as sales increase in the effort to "lower cholesterol."

Most medicines treat the effects of coronary heart disease rather than the cause. Not only are the statins causing bodily harm, but this knowledge of the harm was known by Merck & Co. Why else would Merck file two patents (US 4929437, issued May 20, 1990, and a second patent, US 4933165, issued June 12, 1990) which suggest that **a combination of drug and CoQ10 is necessary? Yet**

doctors more than a decade later do not tell you to take CoQ10 to avoid muscle damage when taking statin drugs.

Another hypocholesterol drug, Baycol, was pulled from the market when it was linked with at least 31 deaths from rhabdomyolysis, which occurs when muscle tissues die and release toxins that can cause organ damage or kidney failure.

Numerous reports over the last decade tell us that statin-related side effects and the magnitude of the potential problem cannot be overstated. Low cholesterol is associated with cancer, depression, criminality, drug abuse, suicide, and more. The use of statins is steadily rising despite a growing understanding of the limited benefit and the increased risks associated with such treatment. Do you know that erectile dysfunction increases in about 50% of men treated with statins?

It is incumbent upon regulatory bodies such as the United States Food and Drug Administration to better monitor the cavalier use of such potentially dangerous drugs based on a flimsy hypothesis. Are statin drugs causing more harm than good? Serious readers should go to www.thincs.org for detailed horror stories.

How great is the problem? Since the statin drug "Crestor" was approved, doctors in more than 73 countries have written more than 22 million prescriptions for this cholesterol-lowering drug. Despite this popularity, some statin ads tell us that the product *"has not been determined to prevent heart disease, heart attacks or strokes."* There are **NO** perceived benefits except lowering cholesterol levels.

One of the most prescribed statins, lipitor, has proven to have side effects. Several comments from the Internet reflect my own experience:

I would not do it [take lipitor] if I were you. It took me over two years to walk normally after 3 months on lipitor 20 mg.

—Larrio

I have a horrific case of peripheral neuropathy from 20 mg of lipitor.

I was on it for only 3 months. I have had the problem for 14 months now. No improvement.

I had memory loss, joint pain in my neck & shoulders, and I was constantly irritated by menial things. All the other symptoms cleared except for the neuropathy.

Trying to find a doctor who believes lipitor causes these side effects is nearly impossible. They keep saying it is idiopathic.

Find a natural alternative. Lose weight, diet, and exercise. Trust me, the side effects from statins are awful!

—MAL

Other stories can be found at www.ravnskov.nu/cholesterol.

Acute coronary events strike nearly 1.4 million Americans annually (www.ravnskov.nu/cholesterol). This includes an estimated 700,000 new coronary events, 500,000 recurrent events, and 175,000 silent first events each year. Adding to the clinical challenge are the facts that while conventional risk factors remain an important means of predicting who is at risk of developing coronary heart disease (CHD), it's unwise to rely on them alone for estimating patient risk. A 2003 evaluation of 122,458 patients enrolled in 14 international trials was meant to underscore the fact that conventional risk factors are still important; yet 20% of men with CHD in these trials had none of the four conventional risk factors analyzed: smoking, hypertension, diabetes, and hyperlipidemia (high cholesterol) (www.ravnskov.nu/cholesterol). Another challenge: Despite the overwhelming effectiveness of HMG-CoA reductase inhibitors (statins) in lipid lowering, 60% to 70% of cardiovascular events continue to occur despite statin therapy. This is in stark contrast to a 1996 prediction that statin therapy might eliminate heart attacks by the year 2000. It should be noted that in the large review of international trials mentioned above, only 34.1% of men with CHD had hyperlipidemia. If the Cholesterol-Heart Hypothesis of atherosclerosis is correct, why do so few CHD patients have hyperlipidemia, and why are so many events still occurring in patients on statin therapy? More intensive statin therapy is not the answer. In the PROVE-IT TIMI-22 study, for example, high-dose statin therapy continued to be associated with a 25% recurrent event rate at 2.5 years (www.ravnskov.nu/cholesterol).

We continue to treat the symptoms/effects and not the problem/cause. **The root cause of the CAD problem is not elevated cholesterol, but the vascular damage that came before signs of high cholesterol.** The initial cause of vascular damage remains the million-dollar question: diet, smoking, infection, chemical environmental stressors, genetic predisposition, or other factors may be at the root of the problem.

The high cholesterol content of an atheroma (artery plaque), the frequent occurrence of myocardial infarction with high serum cholesterol, the extensive arteriosclerotic changes in diseases (nephrosis, myxedema) with high serum cholesterol, and the occurrence of cholesterol deposits in the aorta in some animals fed with cholesterol are the principal arguments for the Cholesterol-Heart Hypothesis of arteriosclerosis. However, many observations contradict this theory. One of the most important observations is that the composition of the atheroma is the same as that of many granulation tissues, *which are generally interpreted as a healing process.* It would seem, therefore, that atheroma tissue could also be interpreted as part of a reparative healing process. Such a new hypothesis could better explain today all the well-known arteriosclerotic changes.

In nature, only a few animals (the higher primates, the guinea pig, and a species of fruit bat) display coronary heart disease, and then only when they are fed a diet lacking adequate amounts of vitamin C. Zookeepers learned the connection between vitamin C and heart health a long time ago. When their gorillas were fed a diet of processed "gorilla chow" instead of a diet rich in vitamin C from fresh fruits and vegetables, they got sick and developed heart disease. Could dosage with vitamin C protect man from heart disease? Recent findings regarding vitamin C have made re-evaluation of this important nutrient imperative. First, vitamin C is now known to be involved in several novel physiological phenomena including stem cell differentiation and respiratory development. These physiological processes likely require significantly high levels of vitamin C. Second, there is a growing recognition that many aging-related diseases, including heart disease, neural degeneration, and cancer, may have a contributing oxidative damage factor that might be reduced by dietary antioxidants such as vitamins C and E.

The role of vitamin C in reducing heart disease episodes needs to be further tested. Perhaps Linus Pauling was correct in suggesting high doses of this vitamin.

The cholesterol level of a bear can be three times as high as a man's, and the bear's heart rate slows down considerably during hibernation. Yet remarkably, bears never show any atherosclerosis nor suffer from stroke. So, what is going on in bears that is missing in humans, apes, guinea pigs, and some fruit bats?

I support a new paradigm that high cholesterol is a response to some injurious agent and is not a cause of the injury. Thus, cholesterol forms part of a protective mechanism. This hypothesis is more compatible with the known facts about the relationship of cholesterol to arteriosclerosis.

Currently, the re-emerging response-to-injury theory on the role of inflammation and infection in atherosclerosis seems to explain many clinical facts not taken into account by other theories. I view elevated cholesterol, C-reactive protein, and Lp(a) for what they really are: the body's dire attempt to save itself. These so-called "bad guys" are just markers of injury, and they proliferate when the body is under stress. The most recent refinement of the Injury Theory proposes that arterial cell wall dysfunction/damage alone is sufficient to initiate atherosclerosis.

In summary, atherosclerosis develops because of a co-existent inflammatory response due to cell injury, proliferation of smooth muscle cells, and finally lipid accumulation in the vessel wall. The critical question is—what caused the initial injury?

Demise of the Cholesterol-Heart Hypothesis

There are currently two main hypotheses to explain the onset and progression of atherosclerotic heart disease. The first—and most vigorously promoted—claims that high cholesterol levels in the bloodstream somehow initiate damage to the artery wall, causing atherosclerosis, as well as increasing the tendency for blood to form artery-blocking clots.

The second theory postulates that atherosclerosis is initiated by direct damage of the artery walls by a number of factors, including smoking, hyperhomocysteinemia, iron overload, copper deficiency, oxidized cholesterol, micro-organisms (bacteria, viruses), and free radical damage that accompanies elevated blood sugar levels. The latter is seen in diabetics, who suffer heart disease at a greatly increased rate compared to non-diabetics.

The utter failure of dietary cholesterol-lowering trials to prevent coronary heart disease, as well as the lack of relationship between the degree of cholesterol lowering and survival, cast doubt on the Cholesterol-Heart theory of heart disease. Depending on the study, high blood cholesterol is unrelated to overall mortality. In fact, high cholesterol predicts greater longevity in the elderly.

Dr. Hans Kaunitz in his papers has reported the following:

> Arteriosclerosis is believed by many to represent the aging process of arteries and to be responsible for the cause-specific deaths at any age in industrialized countries. *The increasing rate of arteriosclerosis is associated with steadily increasing life expectancy.* A report of the average age at

death (AAD) of conditions with prominent arteriosclerosis (ischemic heart disease, myocardial infarction, cerebrovascular disease, "atherosclerosis") was obtained from Vital Statistics of the U.S.A. (Vol. II, Mortality), Section 8:71–195.

Persons above the age of 40 were studied. The arteriosclerosis groups were compared to the "normals" from whom (in addition to the groups with prominent arteriosclerosis) accidents, suicides, homicides, and other "external" causes of death were deducted. In general the arteriosclerosis groups had significantly higher AADs than the "normals." Although arteriosclerosis may exceed its normal function leading to lesions (e.g. myocardial infarction), in the majority of the cases it seems to be a life-prolonging adaptive process which is in line with evolutionary expectations.

This strongly indicates that the Cholesterol-Heart Hypothesis has a weak connection with scientific reality and supports the idea that cholesterol is not the culprit that many think it is.

The New Paradigm: Atherosclerosis as an Inflammatory Disease

Due to their poor understanding of the complex biological properties of the artery wall, researchers active in the first half of the twentieth century looked at atherosclerosis as a simple plumbing problem. If there were too much lipid floating around in the circulation, it would eventually stick to the inside of the arteries; and if this buildup of fat became large enough, blood flow would stop. It was also generally believed that atherosclerosis was an inevitable consequence of aging. There was not much that medicine could do about the aging process.

In the early 1970s, our view about coronary artery disease (CAD) and cholesterol started to change. At that point, a great deal had been learned about the biological functions of vascular cells. Russell Ross, a pathologist working at the University of Washington, suggested that atherosclerosis develops because of the artery wall's response to injury, and that the scarring is caused by a growth factor released from platelets (Ross 1993). This proposal initiated a slow shift in atherosclerosis research, focusing attention on understanding the biology of vascular function, damage, and repair.

The idea that the disease develops in response to some kind of injury and resulting inflammation is becoming more widely accepted by many scientists. A linkage between stress and heart disease is universally accepted. It is known that the stress hormone cortisol can cause chronic inflammation of blood vessels. This inflammation damages artery walls and promotes atherosclerosis. Since inflammation is central to the development of coronary artery disease, markers of inflammation have been tested in respect to heart health. *C-reactive protein (CRP) was found to be the only marker of inflammation that independently predicts the risk of a heart attack.* The CRP test should therefore be added to the screening battery of cholesterol and other lipid tests to detect people at risk for a heart attack.

C-Reactive Protein as an Inflammatory Marker and Risk Factor for CAD

C-reactive protein (CRP) is an acute non-specific phase reactant, released in the body in response to acute injury, infection, or other inflammatory stimuli. In the past few years development of a high-sensitivity assay for CRP has enabled investigation of this marker of systemic inflammation. Atheromatous plaques in diseased arteries typically contain inflammatory cells. Rupture of atheromatous plaque is thought to be the mechanism for acute myocardial infarction. Thus, the release of acute phase reactants as a response to inflammation has been proposed as a potential marker of an "unstable" atheromatous plaque and underlying atherosclerosis.

C-reactive protein is released into the bloodstream each time there is active inflammation in the body, which occurs in response to infection, injury, or various conditions such as arthritis. Evidence is accumulating that atherosclerosis (coronary artery disease, CAD) is initiated by an inflammatory process. The fact that elevated CRP levels are associated more than cholesterol levels with an increased risk of heart attack tends to better support the proposed relationship between inflammation and atherosclerosis than cholesterol levels alone.

Studies have shown a positive association between CRP and coronary artery disease. In a survey of men and women, the prevalence of coronary artery disease increased 1.5-fold for each doubling of CRP level (Boekholdt et al. 2006). This study suggests that in addition to measuring lipid level, CRP may be a better marker of cardiovascular risk than cholesterol.

An article appearing in the November 14, 2002 issue of the *New England Journal of Medicine* confirms that, at least in women, an elevated blood level of CRP is strongly predictive of future cardiovascular events (such as heart attack and stroke). These results came from an analysis of more than 20,000 blood samples taken from women enrolled in the Women's Health Study. This long-term study followed apparently healthy women for a number of years. An earlier (2000) study by Ridker et al. found similar associations.

While elevated CRP levels have been associated with cardiovascular risk in the past, these new reports offer striking evidence that elevated CRP may be a better risk factor than elevated low-density lipoprotein (LDL, "bad") cholesterol levels. Furthermore, high CRP levels may identify high-risk patients who would be "missed" by measuring cholesterol levels alone. In the Women's Health Study, women with low CRP and low cholesterol did well, while those with high CRP and high cholesterol were high risk. Women with either high CRP or high cholesterol also had elevated risk, and those with high CRP but normal cholesterol apparently had a higher risk than those with normal CRP and high LDL cholesterol.

Elevated CRP appears to provide a reasonable explanation for the development of atherosclerosis. To fully characterize an individual's risk of cardiovascular "events," measuring CRP should be added to the list of screening tests. However, the question remains as to what causes the injury/inflammation in the first place.

Certain lifestyle changes including a smarter diet, increased exercise, and the elimination of smoking, excessive weight, and stress can lead to a reduction in CRP levels. While we don't know the best ways to reduce CRP levels, or even whether reducing CRP levels will, in turn, reduce cardiovascular risk, we do know what may raise levels. Smoking in particular elevates the CRP levels. Furthermore, metabolic Syndrome X (Insulin Resistance/Obesity) is associated with high CRP levels. This fact provides us with yet another compelling reason to reduce our weight and to exercise regularly. A common cause of elevated CRP levels is periodontal (gum) disease. Poor oral hygiene has been associated with an increased risk of heart attacks and stroke. In fact, dentists are engaged in studies to see whether an antibiotic gel rubbed on the gums can reduce CRP levels and cardiovascular events. This has been discussed in Chapter 6. A monolaurin paste has been useful in such situations for individuals who have tested it for tooth pain.

Most of the available evidence today suggests that pro-inflammatory cells dominate the atherosclerotic process. The most important challenge is to find the plaque antigen recognized by the T cells. Infectious microorganisms represent one obvious class of candidates. Could it be that bacteria or viruses infect the vascular wall, and that the combined attack of the immune system against both lipids and microorganisms has deleterious effects? Several types of microorganisms have been detected in plaques. Antibody levels against some of these, primarily one called *Chlamydia pneumoniae (C. pneumoniae)*, were increased in subjects suffering from cardiovascular disease.

Exploring the Role of Infection in Atherosclerosis

In many patients, traditional risk factors such as abnormal lipid metabolism, tobacco abuse, hypertension, and diabetes often do not totally account for atherosclerosis. Accumulating evidence suggests that atherosclerosis is an inflammatory disease; therefore, a great deal of attention has been focused on the possibility that infectious agents play a role in the etiology of coronary artery disease.

Epidemiological studies suggest an association between some pathogens and atherosclerosis. Two infectious agents, *C. pneumoniae* and cytomegalovirus, have been detected in human atherosclerotic lesions. Antibodies to *C. pneumoniae* are associated with the risk of premature myocardial infarction (MI) in current and former smokers. Elevated antibody levels to both *C. pneumoniae* and cytomegalovirus confer a higher risk for premature MI, even after adjustment for other risk factors. Doubly seropositive patients also tend to have increased levels of inflammatory markers, including CRP. The issue is not without controversy, and more work needs to be done in this area.

A recent study found that infection with multiple pathogens (bacteria and viruses) could contribute to coronary artery disease by causing endothelial cell injury and resulting inflammation (Vahdat et al. 2007). It has also been suggested that herpes viruses may infect vascular cells, inducing a proinflammatory change in the vessel wall which can, in turn, predispose it to cellular degeneration and atherosclerosis.

The full story remains complex. There are many risk factors associated with vascular disease, including hypertension, chemicals/tobacco, hyperlipidemia, diabetes, immunological factors, and infectious agents such as bacteria and viruses. The majority of these risk factors are present in a relatively small percentage of the population;

by contrast, the herpes virus (60–100%) and the gram-negative bacteria *C. pneumoniae* (50–70%) are ubiquitous in the population.

Traditionally, it is assumed that infectious agents induce disease by tissue damage via secretion of toxins. These toxins may directly or indirectly induce tissue damage and cause release of tissue antigens. Studies support the pathogenesis of vascular disease from the inflammatory component caused by infectious agents. Patients with acute myocardial infarction have long been recognized as having a high plasma concentration or count of markers of inflammation, such as an erythrocyte sedimentation rate, C-reactive protein, fibrinogen, or white blood cell count.

One mechanism of action suggests that an infectious agent from diseased gums or the lungs is taken up by macrophages, transferred to the bloodstream, and finally attacks the arteries. When a macrophage burrows into the wall of a blood vessel to gobble up irritants such as LDL and oxidized LDL, it transfers the infectious agent(s) into the neighboring arterial cells. Infected arterial cells attract more macrophages and other inflammatory responses, such as platelets, and then die. As a result, anti-platelet and endothelial cell antibodies are produced. If this vicious cycle of inflammation continues, it can result in fibrous lesions or plaque formation. When pieces of the plaque break loose, they can start blood clots and cause heart attack.

These findings have direct relevance to the diagnosis and treatment of the many human diseases to which a microbial infection is linked. Fats are therefore important since some saturated and unsaturated lipids are antimicrobial, and cholesterol is necessary for a healthy immune system. In fact, the American College of Cardiology issued a list (Table 9.1) of harmful pathogens as possible bacterial/viral links in the disease process for heart and vascular failure. These pathogens may induce their pathologic responses through one of the above-mentioned mechanisms of action.

TABLE 9.1

List of microorganisms that share similar antigens with human tissue and may induce cardiovascular disease

Human myosin—heart target antigen in cardiovascular disease

Borrelia burgdorferi—the spirochete causing Lyme disease

Treponema pallidum—the causative agent of syphilis

Mycoplasma pneumoniae—non-viral primary, atypical pneumonia

Mycoplasma genitalium—associated with urogenital infection

Mycoplasma fermentans and *M. oralis*—involved in gum disease

Chlamydia pneumoniae—an etiological agent of pneumonia

Helicobacter pylori—associated with duodenal and gastric ulcer

Coxsackie virus—associated with myocarditis

Cytomegalovirus—infection in immuno-compromised individuals

Epstein-Barr virus—infectious mononucleosis and human cancer

Herpes Type-2 virus—associated primarily in human genital infection, and some respiratory problems in cats and horses

Hepatitis A virus—associated with infection of the liver

Streptococcus sanguis and *S. oralis*—periodontal-associated disease

Porphyromonas gingivalis—an aerobic bacteria isolated from pulpal infections involved in gum disease

Due to immunological reactions against these invading microorganisms, high levels of IgG antibodies against bacterial antigens and pathogenic peptides (for example, myosin) are detected in both animal models and human blood. The American College of Cardiology found that, in 890 blood samples, levels of IgG antibodies against some of these bacteria or viruses were significantly higher in 167 patients who later suffered a heart attack or cardiovascular death. Examining 500 blood specimens from patients with cardiovascular disease then comparing them to 500 blood samples of healthy controls confirmed the conclusions of these findings. Subsequently it was found that 33% and 22% of patients versus 9% and 3% of control subjects, respectively, had significant elevations of IgG and IgM antibodies against cardiac myosin and pathogens involved in periodontal and/or cardiovascular disease.

It should be noted that most of the organisms on the above list can be adversely affected by saturated acids or an antimicrobial saturated monoglyceride supplement like Lauricidin. Perhaps adding a daily supplement like Lauricidin to the diet could reduce or eliminate the incidence of heart disease. This hypothesis remains to be studied.

Conclusions

- In inflammatory heart disease of patients without established risk factors, infectious agents play a crucial role.
- Inflammatory heart disease is developed by different mechanisms, including the T-cell-dependent production of autoantibodies against cardiac myosin.

- Early detection of these antibodies is the best indicator of the involvement of infectious agents and inflammation in the sub-population of patients with cardiovascular disease.
- Detection of IgG or IgM antibodies against antigens of infectious agents should be used for determination of the presence of potentially pathogenic organisms.
- Early intervention and eradication of these microorganisms from the oral cavity, lungs, and blood with antibiotic/monolaurin use may improve clinical conditions and quality of life for patients with cardiovascular disease.

Clinicians point out that *if* microbes cause persistent infection in the vessel wall, they could directly promote a proinflammatory, procoagulant, and pro-atherogenic environment.

A paradox is that coronary heart disease morbidity and mortality have been in steady decline in industrialized countries since the 1960s. This decline has been attributed to changes in dietary habits and to a decrease in incidence of conventional risk factors such as smoking and hypertension. One also needs to consider that during this time quick emergency medicine, highly skilled bypass surgery, and intervention with implanted pacemakers and/or defibrillators have made substantial contributions to reduced mortality from coronary heart disease.

Dr. R.C. Meier recently suggested still another alternative explanation: "Could it be that the decline started when tetracycline antibiotics came on the market? This trend has continued after the introduction of macrolides and fluoroquinolones for the treatment of different types of infection. These treatments might have influenced the course of *C. pneumoniae, H. pylori,* and dental infections in affected people. The first preliminary intervention trials with antibiotics in CHD [coronary heart disease] patients gave positive results: azithromycin decreased cardiac events in patients with raised *C. pneumoniae* antibodies. Roxithromycin had similar effects in patients with unstable angina. In both studies, a reduction in inflammation markers was also seen" (Meier 2000).

However, several large-scale prospective antibiotic intervention trials with thousands of patients—such as WIZARD, ACES, and PROVE-IT—have not seen any statistically significant benefits of antibiotic treatment with coronary artery disease patients. At the same time, the clinicians declare that such trials, "even if unsuccessful, will not disprove the *C. pneumoniae* theory, because we do not know the right therapy or even how to find the patients who might benefit most from antimicrobial drugs" (Muhlestein 2002). In addition, antibiotics as well as statins are known to reduce inflammation. Why statins? The mechanism is not only the lowering of cholesterol but perhaps their anti-oxygen effects.

Most researchers acknowledge that the microbial pathogenesis theory for atherosclerosis remains unverified. They conclude, however, that since several of the pathogens linked with atherosclerosis are amenable to treatment, further studies to verify causality are urgently needed.

Cytomegalovirus infection is strongly linked to coronary artery reblockage after angioplasty, and also to accelerated coronary artery disease after cardiac transplantation. New data on this topic are appearing in the literature almost every month. Novel therapeutic management of cardiovascular disease and stroke by monolaurin has the potential to be effective if infection is proven to cause or accelerate CAD.

Current studies provide new insight into the complex mechanisms whereby hyperlipidemia is associated with but is not the cause of progressive atherosclerosis. It is known that physical injury to the endothelial lining of arteries sets off a process (higher cholesterol values) which is probably an attempt at healing the injury, but which unfortunately can lead to atherosclerosis.

Depending on the validity of this old/new view of atherosclerosis, monolaurin could play a major role in a healthy lifestyle. Not only has it been shown that monolaurin can affect most microorganisms implicated in heart disease, but its daily use would give protection without the danger of forming resistant organisms. Because of its complete lack of toxicity and side effects, monolaurin is a great gift from nature for wellness and self-healing. Advocates believing in this approach need as soon as possible to support clinical trials.

CHAPTER 10

Benign Prostatic Hyperplasia

Benign (non-cancerous) enlargement of the prostate, known as benign prostatic hyperplasia (BPH for short), is the most common prostate problem in men. As men age, almost all of them will develop some enlargement of the prostate. Overall, the number of men with BPH increases progressively with age. By age 60, 50% of men will have some signs of BPH. By age 85, 90% of men will have signs of the condition. About one third of these men will develop symptoms that require treatment (statistics from the American Urological Association Education and Research, Inc., 2003).

However, BPH and prostate cancer have similar symptoms, and a man with BPH may have undetected cancer at the same time. To help detect prostate cancer in its early stages, annual screening of prostate-specific antigen (PSA) should start at age 50. For men who are at high risk, such as African Americans and men with a family history of prostate cancer, screening should begin at about age 45. Men at an even higher risk, who have several relatives with a history of prostate cancer at an early age, could begin testing at age 40. There is no agreement as to the value of the PSA test, but it represents a simple window to prostate health. The reader is encouraged to review the following Internet website: www.majidali.com/psa_clinical_value_prostate_cancer.

While drugs are available for this problem, the natural supplement saw palmetto is widely used for relief from the swelling and discomfort of an enlarged prostate gland. Chemical analysis of this plant indicates that monolaurin is one of its most active components because of the inhibition of the enzyme 5 alpha-reductase, which is responsible for the conversion of testosterone (T) to its more potent androgen dihydrotestosterone (DHT). This steroid has been implicated in androgen-dependent diseases such as benign prostatic hyperplasia, prostate cancer, acne, and androgenic alopecia.

For many centuries, benign prostatic hyperplasia (nonmalignant enlargement of the prostate gland, also called benign prostatic hypertrophy) has undoubtedly been an important cause of the urinary difficulties observed in elderly men. The condition was only recognized as such in the last hundred years. Benign prostatic hyperplasia (BPH) is a common condition. Eighty-eight percent of autopsy specimens in men over 80 have histological BPH. It is the reason for the most common surgical procedure in elderly men. Three men in ten ultimately may require surgery for this condition. It is estimated that 50% of men over 55 years of age have urinary problems. Although labeled benign, this swelling of the prostate was a common cause of death in elderly men up to two or three decades ago. Improved medical care has seen dramatic declines in this aspect of BPH, and today treatment choices in BPH are largely determined by considerations of quality-of-life. Despite such a common occurrence, little is known with any certainty about the epidemiology of BPH. (Epidemiology is the study of the origin and development of a particular disease.) The incidence, even the population prevalence, is difficult to determine for a variety of reasons. Case-control studies, the most commonly employed design in epidemiology, are problematic in that a control group may be difficult to define in view of the likelihood that a large proportion of these may have undiagnosed BPH.

Against this background, knowledge of the prostate in the general population was sought in an international survey and found to be poor (Boyle 1994). Although most men are aware of its existence, very few could correctly identify the function of the gland. Men tended to discuss urination problems with their doctors not when a symptom developed, but when that symptom became bothersome. Given the large increase in the number of males reaching older ages, it is clear that BPH will continue to have substantial and increasing influence in terms of morbidity, mortality, and health costs. Before the end of the present century, the life expectancy of a male at birth will exceed 80 years in many of the developed countries. This means that one man in every two born can expect to reach an age at which he will have an 88% chance of having a prostate with morphological BPH. The need is clear for high-quality epidemiological information and consequent increased prospects for prevention. Following is an explanation of the problem and possible solutions, including a solution that is based on healthy saturated fats, like monolaurin, in one's diet.

The Prostate Gland

The prostate is a walnut-sized gland that forms part of the male reproductive system. The gland is made of two lobes, or regions, enclosed by an outer layer of tissue. The prostate is located in front of the rectum and just below the bladder. The prostate also surrounds the urethra, the duct through which urine passes out of the body. Scientists do not know all the prostate's functions. One of its main roles, though, is to squeeze fluid into the urethra as the sperm moves through during sexual climax. This fluid, which helps make up semen, energizes the sperm. Normally the pH of semen is alkaline because of the seminal vesicle secretion. An alkaline pH protects the sperm from the acidity of the vaginal fluid.

As mentioned, it is common for the prostate gland to become enlarged as a man ages. The prostate goes through two main periods of growth. The first occurs early in puberty, when the gland doubles in size. At around age 25, it begins to grow again. This second growth phase often results in BPH years later.

Though the prostate continues to grow during most of a man's life, the enlargement doesn't usually cause problems until late in life. BPH rarely causes symptoms before age 40, but more than half of men in their sixties and as many as 90% in their seventies and eighties have some symptoms of BPH.

As the prostate enlarges, the surrounding capsule stops it from expanding, causing the gland to press against the urethra like a clamp on a garden hose. The bladder wall becomes thicker and irritable. The bladder begins to contract, even when it contains small amounts of urine, causing urination to be more frequent. As the bladder weakens, it loses the ability to empty itself and urine remains behind. This narrowing of the urethra and partial emptying of the bladder associated with BPH causes much of the difficulty or pain during urination.

Many people feel uncomfortable talking about the prostate, since the gland plays a role in both sex and urination. Still, prostate enlargement is as common a part of aging as gray hair. As life expectancy rises, so does the occurrence of BPH. In the United States alone, it is not clear whether certain groups face a greater risk of getting BPH. Studies over the years suggest that BPH occurs more often among married men than single men, and it is more common in the United States and Europe than in other parts of the world. These findings have been debated, and no definite information on risk factors exists.

Symptoms of BPH

Many symptoms of BPH stem from obstruction of the urethra and gradually declining bladder function, which result in incomplete emptying of the bladder. The symptoms of BPH vary, but the most common ones involve changes or problems with urinating, such as the following:

a. a hesitant, interrupted, weak stream;

b. urgency and leaking or dribbling;

c. more frequent urination, especially at night.

The size of the prostate does not always determine how severe the obstruction or symptoms will be. Some men with greatly enlarged glands have little obstruction symptoms, while other men with less enlarged glands have more blockage problems. Sometimes a man may not know he has any obstruction until he suddenly finds himself unable to urinate at all. Taking over-the-counter cold or allergy medicines can trigger this condition, called acute urinary retention. Such medicines contain a decongestive drug that may as a side effect prevent the bladder opening from relaxing and allowing urine to empty. Alcohol, cold temperatures, or a long immobility can also bring on partial urinary retention.

Severe BPH can cause serious problems over time. Urine retention and strain on the bladder can lead to urinary tract infections, bladder or kidney damage, or incontinence. If the bladder is permanently damaged, drug treatment for BPH is ineffective. When BPH is found in its earlier stages, there is a lower risk of developing such complications.

How BPH Occurs

The cause of BPH is not well understood. It has been known for centuries that the condition occurs mainly in older men, and that it doesn't develop in males whose testes are removed before puberty. For this reason, some researchers believe that factors regarding aging of the testes may spur the development of BPH. Throughout their lives, men produce testosterone, an important male hormone, and small amounts of estrogen, a female hormone. As men age, the amount of testosterone in the blood decreases, and this leaves a greater proportion of estrogen. Studies with animals have suggested that BPH may occur because the higher amount of estrogen within the gland increases the activity of substances that promote cell growth.

Another theory focuses on dihydrotestosterone (DHT), a substance derived from testosterone in the prostate, which affects its growth. Most animals lose the ability to produce DHT as they age. However, some research indicates that despite a drop in the blood's testosterone level of older men, they continue to produce and accumulate levels of DHT in the prostate. This accumulation of DHT encourages the greater growth of cells. Scientists have also noted that men who do not produce DHT do not develop BPH.

Although human benign prostatic hyperplasia is the most common tumor in men, its etiology remains unclear. At present, it is widely accepted that BPH is under the endocrine control of the testes and strongly associated with aging. Therefore, in the human prostate we describe the impact of aging on the activity of various testosterone-metabolizing enzymes as well as on the endogenous testosterone and estrogen levels.

Among all testosterone-metabolizing enzymes within the human prostate, 5 alpha-reductase is the most powerful. This enzyme, which converts testosterone to dihydrotestosterone, undergoes a significant increase with aging. Even with aging the 5 alpha-reductase maintains its role as the most dominant androgen-metabolizing enzyme. This could be of pathogenetic importance for BPH development. The inhibition of 5 alpha-reductase activity by the drug finasteride (Prosper) leads to a size reduction in BPH. Thus it has been concluded that one of the major triggering factors for BPH is dihydrotestosterone (DHT), which is produced from testosterone by the action of the enzyme 5 alpha-reductase. Compounds that inhibit this enzyme can generally be expected to have a beneficial effect on BPH.

Nutriceutical Treatment of BPH

In 1990, 61 million Americans were estimated to have used some form of alternative medicine to treat all forms of ailments, spending at least $27 billion a year. Visits to practitioners of alternative medicine have also risen sharply, from 427 million in 1990 to 629 million in 1997. Today alternative medicine is a $30 billion industry (Krizner 2005). Those figures stand in marked contrast with visits to establishment doctors, which were reduced. In a keynote address at the International Complementary & Natural Healthcare Expo in Los Angeles in 2005, Dr. David Eisenberg (Center for Alternative Medicine Research and Education at the Beth Israel Deaconess Medical Center in Boston) said, "These numbers are the strongest message that the market can deliver to the medical establishment."

People seeking alternative medical care are often concerned about the serious side effects and high cost of prescription drugs and are thus interested in treating a condition with more natural substances. One of the more common plant extracts used for BPH is obtained from the saw palmetto. Western knowledge of the benefits of saw palmetto *(Serenoa repens;* also known as the dwarf American palm, cabbage palm, fan palm, scrub palm, Serenoa, sabal, and *Sabal serrulata)* can be traced back to the early 1700s. It was observed that the aborigines of the Florida peninsula depended largely upon the berries, which they used to treat atrophy of the testes, impotence, inflammation of the prostate, and low libido in men, and as a general tonic to nourish the body. Other historical uses have included the treatment of infertility and underdeveloped breasts in women, to increase lactation, and to lessen the effects of painful menstrual periods. Saw palmetto has also been used as an anti-inflammatory, appetite stimulant, and a tonic and expectorant for mucous membranes, particularly the bronchial passages. It has been marketed as an aphrodisiac for both men and women and was once called "the sex pill of the '90s." Today, however, the product is mainly used for the treatment of conditions associated with BPH.

Because of the significant risks and complications of surgery and the high cost of the procedure, World Health Organization guidelines recommend finasteride or alpha-blocker drugs as treatment options for men with bothersome symptoms. Finasteride therapy reduces the size of the hyperplastic prostate gland by more than 20%, improves the urinary flow rate, and reduces the symptoms associated with bladder outlet obstruction. Although statistically significant, results obtained with finasteride are just slightly better than placebo. Finasteride is well tolerated by most men, and adverse events are rare. However, it decreases serum PSA (prostate-specific antigen) by 50%. PSA is a biochemical marker for malignant prostatic cancer. It is essential for elderly males to have this test to carefully monitor their health and exclude prostate cancer before initiation and during therapy for BPH.

The drug permixon is another lipid extract of the saw palmetto plant and is a complex mixture of various compounds. A form of the drug has been used in treatment of prostatic conditions dating back to the 1800s. In controlled clinical trials, oral administration of 160 mg of permixon twice daily for one to three months was generally superior to placebo in improving subjective symptoms. The frequency of nocturnal urination was reduced by 33 to 74%, while urinary frequency during the day decreased by 43%, and peak urinary flow rate increased by 26 to 50%. Corresponding values for placebo were 13 to 39% (Gerber et al. 2001).

A summary conclusion indicates that the *Serenoa repens* supplement is well tolerated and has greater efficacy than placebo and similar efficacy to the drug finasteride in improving symptoms of BPH. Although there is a need for further comparative studies, available data indicate that *Serenoa repens* is a useful alternative to finasteride in the treatment of men with BPH.

Since extracts from fruit of *Serenoa repens* are used in the treatment of human benign prostatic hyperplasia, it is of interest whether this phytopharmacon has any influence on the androgen metabolism in the human prostate. It was found that the crude extract of the plant inhibited 5 alpha-reductase activities in the epithelium and stroma cells of human BPH. The mean inhibition was 29% and 45%, respectively (Shimada et al. 1997). Table 10.1 lists the components in saw palmetto and their effect on 5 alpha-reductase of the prostate gland.

TABLE 10.1

% Inhibition of 5 alpha-reductase

Fatty Acid	Epithelium	Stroma
Lauric acid C12	51	42
Myristic acid C14	43	34
Palmitic acid C16	2	0
Oleic acid C18:1	5	0
Phytosterols	15	10
CHO, AA, and Polysaccharides	0	0

In vitro studies resulting in this chart suggested that the saw palmetto's lipid extract has an inhibitory effect on 5 alpha-reductase in both the epithelium and stroma cells of the human prostate. The strong inhibitory effect of saturated fatty acids (lauric C12 and myristic C14 acid) was dose-dependent. As the chart shows, the maximal inhibition in the epithelium and stroma tissue by the saturated fatty acid, lauric acid, was 51% and 42%, respectively. Other fractions of the extract, consisting mainly of phytosterols, showed a mean inhibition of 5 alpha-reductase in the epithelium (15%) and stroma (10%). Finally, the water-soluble subfraction containing carbohydrates (CHO), amino acids (AA), and polysaccharides showed no inhibitory effect.

Additional fractionations with 95% ethanol extract (FOO5) of the powdered dried berries of saw palmetto *(Serenoa repens)* were tested in the laboratory (Shimada et al. 1997). This led to the isolation of two saturated monoglycerides: monolaurin/Lauricidin (fraction 1) and monomyristin (fraction 2). The monolaurin was the most active fraction. Both compounds also showed moderate biological activities against renal (A-498) and pancreatic (PACA-2) human tumor cells; borderline cytotoxicity was exhibited against human prostatic (PC-3) cells (see Table 10.2).

Inhibition of 5 Alpha-Reductase

The 5 alpha-reductase enzyme found in the human scalp has been compared with the enzyme found in the prostate gland. Again, the 5 alpha-reductase catalyzes the reduction of testosterone to dihydrotestosterone in both tissues. The scalp reductase has a broad pH

TABLE 10.2

Bioactivities of fractions F005, 1 and 2

	BSLT(a)	A-498(b)	PC-3(c)	PACA-2(d)
F005 (MeOH)	79.9	31.5	35.7	29.9
Monolaurin (1)	79.2	3.77	23.28	2.33
Monomyristin (2)	53.3	3.5	8.84	1.87
Adriamycin (e)		0.01	0.01	0.04

(a) Brine shrimp lethality test; LC50 values are in µg/mL. (b) Kidney carcinoma. (c) Prostate adenocarcinoma. (d) Pancreas carcinoma. (e) Adriamycin, a DNA-interacting drug widely used in chemotherapy, was utilized as a positive control standard for the BST test.

optimum centered at pH 7.0. This is distinctly different from the pH optimum of 5.5 observed with the prostatic form of the enzyme. These observations indicate that two different forms of 5 alpha-reductase may exist. The scalp reductase was similar to 5 alpha-reductase II, one of the two isoenzymes found in human prostate.

Lipid extracts of saw palmetto seem to have an effect on retarding the hair loss process in androgenetic alopecia (baldness). It is known that the increased transformation of testosterone into dihydrotestosterone is the reason for this hair loss. Finasteride, an inhibitor of 5 alpha-reductase (II) that is used to reduce the effects of benign prostatic hyperplasia, inhibits conversion of testosterone to dihydrotestosterone, resulting in a decrease in serum and scalp dihydrotestosterone levels believed to be pathogenic in androgenetic alopecia.

A study by Morganti et al. (personal communication) showed that a topical treatment performed with a lotion containing an extract from the saw palmetto produced a desired increase in hair numbers of 17% starting within week 10. This increase continued steadily throughout the study and reached 27% at week 50. This result is undoubtedly due to the activity of the 5 alpha-reductase inhibition by saw palmetto extracts.

While I have received testimonial reports that taking monolaurin leads to a stoppage of hair loss, no specific study has been carried out to date to substantiate these testimonials. However, from the known inhibitory effects of monolaurin on 5 alpha-reductase, it seems highly plausible that this supplement may be useful to reduce or prevent hair loss, as well as minimize the undesirable symptoms of BPH.

CHAPTER 11

Nutriceutical Treatment for Gastric Ulcers

For many years, the cause of gastric ulcer disease was widely believed to be associated with a disturbance in the balance between the presence of noxious agents in the stomach and mucosal protective mechanisms. As a result, much of the early research on ulcer disease focused on the role of gastric acid in the genesis of peptic ulceration. While suppression of acid production brings relief in healing acute ulcers, the recurrence rate during the first year can be as high as 90%. This indicates that such treatment is effective in healing the ulcers but not in curing the disease. The more modern approach is to consider the problem of ulcers to be due to an infection rather than to stomach acid imbalance alone. Because gastric ulcers may be an infectious problem, the non-toxic monolaurin, a natural antimicrobial, should be an ideal candidate for keeping people healthy and for self-healing.

The New Paradigm for Gastric Disease

Few of the early investigations of gastric disease explored an infectious etiology until 1984 when Marshall and Warren described the isolation of gram-negative spiral-shaped bacteria from biopsy specimens obtained from human subjects with gastritis and peptic ulcers. These investigators later identified this organism as *Campylobacter pylori.* Subsequent studies have confirmed that this bacterium, currently referred to as *Helicobacter pylori,* is a major etiologic agent in chronic diffuse superficial (type B) gastritis and gastroduodenal ulcer disease. Evidence to support such an association was provided by studies in human volunteers that were challenged with *H. pylori.* A similar association between gastric diseases and spiral organisms was found in the stomachs of laboratory animals. While *H. pylori* infection is extremely common in both children and adults in scores of countries throughout the world, many individuals remain infected for years without developing symptoms of gastritis or ulcer disease. Reports have also appeared regarding a possible association between *H. pylori* infection and the development of gastric carcinoma.

Histological studies have determined that *H. pylori* colonize the mucous layer overlying the epithelial cells in the stomach and do not appear to invade gastric tissue. While many antimicrobial agents exist with good activity *in vitro* against *H. pylori,* evaluation of single agents in clinical trials has not resulted in consistent long-term eradication of the organism from the upper gastrointestinal tract. Results from trials with two or more antibiotics, however, indicate that eradication of *H. pylori* is associated with both the resolution of gastritis and significant decreases in relapse rate of duodenal ulcers compared to treatment with antacids alone. The most effective treatment regimen currently available involves a two-week course of triple therapy consisting of a bismuth compound together with metronidazole and either tetracycline or amoxicillin. However, there are problems associated with the triple-therapy approach to eradicating *H. pylori,* such as non-compliance due to the taste and number of tablets and capsules needed; the onset of side effects such as nausea, diarrhea, and dizziness; and ineffectiveness against antibiotic-resistant strains of *H. pylori.* Other similar approaches have been tried, but collectively these studies indicate that better ways are needed of achieving consistent long-term eradication of *H. pylori.*

The antimicrobial properties of various free fatty acids and fatty acid esters such as monolaurin have been previously discussed. Studies have confirmed that both free fatty acids and monoglycerides are capable of inhibiting the growth of both gram-negative and gram-positive types of bacteria. Susceptibility of various bacteria to inactivation by specific fatty acids may be a factor in regulating the different species of bacteria that colonize the various niches in skin as well as the respiratory and gastrointestinal tracts.

Most investigations of the antimicrobial properties of free fatty acids and monoglycerides have used *in vitro* models to evaluate the inhibitory effects of short-chain and long-chain saturated and monounsaturated fatty acids; clinical studies have not been done on their inhibitory properties. Results from *in vitro* studies have led experts to reach the following conclusions with regard to fatty acid structure-activity relationships.

1. In general, free fatty acid sensitivity is considered a characteristic of gram-positive bacteria, although a few gram-negative bacteria are also sensitive.

2. Gram-negative bacteria are affected primarily by very short-chain free fatty acids (C10 or less).

3. Yeasts/fungi are affected by short-chain fatty acids (C10 or less).

It was no surprise to learn from the report of Petschow et al. (1996) that fatty acids and monoglycerides containing C8–C12 fatty acids were effective in inhibiting the gram-negative bacterial pathogen *Helicobacter* (Table 11.1). All Helicobacter species capable of causing gastric problems such as dyspepsia, ulcers, and carcinoma are affected. At the present time *H. pylori* is most commonly associated with such gastric problems.

TABLE 11.1

Bacterial activity of medium-chain fatty acids and monoglycerides for *H. pylori*

FAs or MGs	Conc. (mM)	Change in no. of viable % *H. pylori* cells $\log_{10}$ CFU/ml	
Caprylic acid (C8)	1	-0.05 ±0.05	NS
Capric acid (C10)	1	-0.40 ±0.56	NS
Lauric acid (C12)	1	-4.07 ±1.24	(98.99%)[A]
Monocaprylin (C8)	1	0.01 ±0.01	NS
Monocaprin (C10)	1	-4.59 ±0.42	(99.99%)[A]
Monolaurin (C12)	1	-4.59 ±0.41	(99.99%)[A]

NS—Not Significant
[A]—Significantly different from the controls

Healing of Gastric Ulcers

The epithelial cells of the stomach and duodenum are normally protected from the damaging effects of gastric acid by a balancing mechanism of acid and mucosal resistance. If an imbalance occurs, peptic ulcers may result. Traditional teaching emphasized the importance of acid (and pepsin) as the cause of this imbalance; however, it is clear that acid alone is not the only important factor in the pathogenesis of peptic ulcers. Epidemiological data indicate an association between *H. pylori* infection and the subsequent development of peptic ulcers and gastric carcinoma.

In the treatment of *H. pylori*-positive duodenal and gastric ulcer, eradication of the infection prevents ulcer relapse, effectively curing the disease. The use of *H. pylori* therapy in non-ulcer dyspepsia remains controversial, and further studies are required. Despite strong circumstantial evidence linking *H. pylori* and gastric cancer, it is premature to advocate *H. pylori* therapy for primary prevention of gastric cancer. Triple therapy (bismuth, metronidazole, and tetracycline) can eradicate *H. pylori* in more than 90% of cases. However, as mentioned, this multidrug regimen is not ideal because of side effects, possible non-compliance, and doubtful efficacy against metronidazole-resistant infection.

Another approach is desperately needed. A group of food-grade nutrients that are antimicrobial may fill this need. These are saturated fatty acids and their corresponding saturated esters (monoglycerides). In laboratory tests, incubation of *H. pylori* with saturated monoglycerides ranging in carbon chain length from C8 to C12 caused reduction in the number of viable bacteria (Table 11.1). Less bactericidal activity was observed with C9, C15, and C16 monoglycerides. In comparison, lauric acid (C12:0) was the only medium-chain saturated fatty acid with the highest bactericidal activity against *H. pylori*. Higher levels of monoglycerides and fatty acids were required for bactericidal activity when added to foods where the presence of protein was high. It was also found that the frequency of spontaneous development of resistance to *H. pylori* was elevated for metronidazole and tetracycline but not for monolaurin (Lauricidin). Collectively, the data demonstrate that medium-chain monoglycerides and lauric acid rapidly inactivate *H. pylori.* As opposed to antibiotics, these non-toxic lipids have a relatively low frequency of spontaneous development of resistance to their bactericidal activity. Monolaurin, like vitamins, needs to be taken daily for better health and self-healing.

Although a number of studies have shown that various fatty acids and monoglycerides have bactericidal properties *in vitro,* the role of these compounds *in vivo* has only been investigated since 1998. A study by Petschow et al. in that year evaluated the antibacterial properties of medium-chain monoglycerides and fatty acids for different bacterial enteropathogens. *In vitro* bacterial killing assay and an *in vivo* model of intestinal colonization were studied. Incubation of test bacteria with medium-chain monoglycerides for four hours led to 100- to 10,000-fold reductions in numbers of viable cells of *Vibrio cholerae, Salmonella typhi, Shigella sonnei,* and enterotoxigenic *Escherichia coli.*

The ability of dietary monoglycerides to reduce or eliminate bacterial colonization of the intestinal tract was evaluated in mice predisposed to bacterial colonization by treatment with streptomycin. These test subjects are referred to as STR+ mice. Treated with streptomycin, mice were challenged intragastrically with *V. cholerae* and given monocaprin (C10:0 saturated monoglyceride) either concurrently or as part of the daily diet. Control mice without monoglycerides and challenged with *V. cholerae* showed high numbers of bacteria in gastrointestinal contents by one hour after administration. Concurrent administration of *V. cholerae* and monocaprin (2.5

mg/ml) caused a greater than 1000-fold reduction in numbers of *V. cholerae* recovered from the gastrointestinal tracts of mice. These results suggest that dietary monoglycerides might prevent intestinal colonization by bacterial enteropathogens if administered prior to or at the time of exposure. Monoglycerides seemed to have little effect on established intestinal infections. This is why taking monolaurin daily is recommended (like the use of vitamins) for well-being and not treatment of acute problems. Monolaurin may represent an essential component for a wellness diet.

A study carried out by Preuss et al. (2005) compared the effect of an antibiotic (vancomycin), oil of oregano, and monolaurin on *Staphylococcus aureus* infection in mice. The control mice died in 10 days. The result after 30 days indicated that monolaurin was as effective as the antibiotic, i.e., 50% survival. The oregano group was similar but less (43%). All 50% in the monolaurin group were cured since *S. aureus* could not be cultured from the survivors.

These two reports using saturated monoglycerides lend confirmation that observations derived from test-tube experiments with Lauricidin could be translated to favorable clinical outcomes. This gives further credibility to testimonials received from users of Lauricidin.

Human Clinical Study

In addition to these animal studies, a small human trial has been carried out to determine if these animal experiments are relevant to human clinical studies. The first clinical trial (1998) of monolaurin took place with fifteen HIV-infected patients reporting regularly at the San Lazaro Hospital (Manila, Philippines). Prior to this trial, these patients did not receive any anti-HIV medication. They were randomly assigned to one of three treatment groups: 2.4g monolaurin TID (3x daily), 7.2g monolaurin TID, and 15ml TID of coconut oil daily for six months. The San Lazaro Hospital Team was led by Eric Tayag, MD, and Conrado Dayrit, MD. I was hired (1998 and 1999) as a consultant to the project. Viral, CD4, and CDS counts, complete blood counts, blood lipids, and tests for liver and kidney functions were done at the beginning of the study and after three and six months of treatment. One patient in the 7.2g TID monolaurin group had a viral load that was too low to count (thus excluded from the trial study).

By the third month, seven of the patients (50%) showed reduced viral load, and by the sixth month nine out of thirteen patients (4/5 receiving 2.4g monolaurin, 2/4 receiving 7.2g monolaurin, and 3/4 receiving coconut oil) had a lowered viral count.

Three patients developed AIDS on the third month of therapy when their CD4 count dropped below 200. One patient in the coconut oil group died two weeks after the study was concluded. The other two AIDS patients were in the 2.4g monolaurin group. One recovered fully on the sixth month, and the other showed a rapid return towards normal CD4 and CD8 counts.

There were no serious side effects observed in any group during the study. Politics and a lack of money prevented further study. The study did encourage me to do further work on my own. Today this is reflected in the many testimonials on the health and self-healing benefits of Lauricidin (see Chapter 13) and the clinical studies that are currently underway.

CHAPTER 12

Reflections on Fifty Years of Research on Saturated Fats and Cholesterol

It used to be that even considering the possibility of an alternative to the Cholesterol-Heart Hypothesis, let alone researching it, was tantamount to quackery by association. Now a small but growing minority of establishment researchers has come to take seriously the flaws that exist in the Cholesterol-Heart Hypothesis. In this book, I have presented to the reader a large amount of scientific evidence showing that elevated cholesterol is *associated* with heart disease but is not a *cause* of heart disease. Recent emphasis on inflammatory markers like C-reactive protein seems to indicate that this marker is more reliable than cholesterol levels in "predicting" heart/vascular problems.

I have also shown that saturated fats are not all the same and that they are definitely not all bad. In fact, some of them are essential for good health and self-healing. As I have stressed earlier, the word "saturated" should be preceded by an adjective, the three adjectives being short-, medium-, and long-chain (saturated fats). Each saturated fat has unique properties and should be distinguished according to its structure.

Unsaturated fats are always mentioned as monounsaturated or polyunsaturated. The sub-classes of polyunsaturated fats are readily known as omega-3 and omega-6. Why have not the saturated fats been given this same distinction? Politics, not science.

As discussed in these pages, medium-chain saturated fats are excellent antimicrobial agents. They seem to be effective against bacteria, yeast/fungi, and even viruses. Their lack of toxicity and failure to induce resistant organisms make them unique biocides.

Medium-chain saturated fats have other desirable properties as well. Certain saturated fatty acids are needed for important cell-signaling functions and proper protein/enzyme activity. The addition of saturated C12, C14, or C16 fatty acids to proteins is necessary for proper functioning of the protein.

Even some long-chain saturated fatty acids have been shown to reduce heart lesions in animals given unsaturated rapeseed oil. (A discussion can be found at www.nexusmagazine.com/articles/canola.html.) Among the food fats tested, the one found to have the best proportion of saturated fat is lard. This is the very fat that people are warned against using under any circumstances, yet its monounsaturated fat content is high (47%), similar to olive oil (76%).

The complex way in which dietary fats interact is not well understood. Fats are not just inert metabolic substances that have calories; they have wide-ranging metabolic effects in the body, and these effects—singularly and collectively—are different for different kinds of fats.

Reviews by Ascherio (2002) and Ravnskov (1998, 2002) of studies that linked dietary cholesterol, fats, and high serum cholesterol with atherosclerosis and cardiovascular disease aptly pointed out that **the results of the epidemiologic and experimental studies are inconclusive or even contradictory. After more than fifty years of research, there is no evidence that consuming a diet low in saturated fat *or* maintaining low cholesterol blood levels prolong life. Some available data indicate that high cholesterol levels in older populations actually lead to greater longevity.**

It is difficult to explain away the fact that during the period of life in which most cardiovascular disease occurs and from which most people die (and most of us die from cardiovascular disease), high cholesterol occurs most often in people with the *lowest mortality.*

To the public and the medical community I say, "We need an oil change for better health."

A News Flash!
From *The New York Times*
December 3, 2006

End of Drug Trial Is a Big Loss for Pfizer and Heart Patients

The news came to Pfizer's chief scientist, Dr. John L. LaMattina. The company's most promising experimental drug, intended to treat heart disease, actually caused an increase in deaths and heart problems. Within hours, Pfizer, the world's largest drug maker, told more than 100 trial investigators to stop giving patients the drug, called "torcetrapib." Pfizer announced that it had pulled the plug on the medicine entirely, turning the company's nearly 1 billion dollar investment in it into a total loss. Scientists had seen torcetrapib as the vanguard of a new wave of medicines that would give physicians new ways to reduce heart disease by raising "good cholesterol" (HDL). Pfizer had been three years into a late-phase clinical trial of torcetrapib involving 15,000 patients.

Not only were there 31 more deaths among the people taking torcetrapib, but side effects were seen in the number of patients suffering heart failure and other problems, giving the company no choice but to stop development.

Pfizer's decision to abandon torcetrapib throws into question the theory that using drugs to raise "good cholesterol" [HDL] will benefit patients. Some scientists worry that the drugs cause the body to produce a form of HDL that may actually be harmful.

This news report is another example of failure in the attempt to prove the validity of the Cholesterol-Heart Hypothesis.

As in war, progress is proclaimed with pomp, while defeats are whispered if reported at all. However, the body of contradictory evidence to the Cholesterol-Heart Hypothesis is readily available to those who want the truth.

The simple bottom-line message of this book is that *all fats* are good when eaten in moderation and balanced in terms of their saturation, monounsaturation, and polyunsaturation content. A suggested balanced and healthy, low-calorie diet would include a fat combination of 25% medium-chain saturated;

57% omega-9 monounsaturated; 3% omega-3; and 15% omega-6. The fat combinations should be included with a low quantity of carbohydrate and modest amounts of protein.

Lauricidin, the medium-chain saturated C12 monoglyceride, was discovered from our initial and original research on lipids. This food-grade saturated lipid, found in low concentration in natural products, is now available as a family and pet supplement for good health and self-healing at www.Lauricidin.com.

For more verification of my point of view I recommend three books:

The Cholesterol Myths: Exposing the Fallacy that Saturated Fat and Cholesterol Cause Heart Disease by Uffe Ravnskov (2000).

The Great Cholesterol Con: Why Everything You've Been Told About Cholesterol, Diet, and Heart Disease Is Wrong by Anthony Colpo (2006).

Prevention of Coronary Heart Disease from the Cholesterol Hypothesis to ω6/ω3 Balance. Contributions by Okuyama, H. (Nagoya); Ichikawa, Y. (Nagoya); Sun, Y. (Dalian); Hamazaki, T. (Toyama); Lands, W.E.M. (College Park, MD), 2007.

Also, read an interesting article, "What if It's All Been a Big Fat Lie?" by Gary Taubes, *New York Times Magazine,* July 7, 2002.

For those of you with Internet access, go to www.thincs.org for fuller disclosures on the myths of cholesterol and saturated fats.

CHAPTER 13

Testimonials

This section is provided as an ad hoc "field report" from people ingesting the high-grade monolaurin product known as Lauricidin, an essential food supplement developed for optimal health and self-healing. The letters and emails have been edited slightly for punctuation and consistency with the rest of the book, but the message has not been altered.

Lauricidin is *not* a drug. Lauricidin achieves its remarkable effects by bring "biochemical balance" to the body, thus allowing the body to heal itself. This is evident from the success stories and the many health professionals who recommend the product to their patients.

These testimonials are unsolicited and uncompensated. The FDA has not evaluated any structure-function statements concerning Lauricidin. This product is not intended to diagnose, treat, cure, or prevent any disease.

The above disclaimer is a requirement of the U.S. Food and Drug Administration, though obviously a food-grade monolaurin product is intended to be taken for health benefits! Many people do claim that it cures and/or prevents various ailments.

My personal experiences and those reported to me suggest that the saturated lipid supplement Lauricidin should become a significant part of a daily healthy diet, much like vitamins.

Professional Endorsement
of Lauricidin

Larry King, CNN Transcript Interview
with Dr. Andrew Weil, MD

CALLER: What do you do for genital herpes?

WEIL: For genital herpes, there are pharmaceutical drugs that suppress it that are effective. They have to be taken all the time and they are expensive. There is a natural product that I'd recommend experimenting with—it's called Lauricidin. I looked this up on the Internet. It's a fatty acid [ester] which is non-toxic. There are some very good clinical reports that it significantly shortens attacks and lowers the frequency of attacks.

John E. Upledger, DO, OMM

Over the past few years we have often recommended the oral administration of Lauricidin for patients/clients as a complement to our one-on-one, hands-on treatment. It is our opinion that Lauricidin has been an effective complement to our work. We have seen these positive effects in patients ranging in diagnosis from viral encephalitis, to reflexive sympathetic dystrophy, to learning-disabled and autistic children. We have not conducted a controlled study, but we have seen a large number of anecdotal cases wherein Lauricidin seemed to be quite helpful. Insofar as Lauricidin has not shown us any adverse clinical reactions, and it is a very low-cost nutritional supplement, we shall continue to use it at The Upledger Institute HealthPlex.

Christopher Scipio, ND

I am not in allopathic medicine so I don't conduct studies, but as a holistic health professional I can absolutely say that my success rate in greatly reducing the severity, duration, and frequency of herpes outbreaks has vastly improved since adding Lauricidin to my protocol.

I am writing a book on the holistic treatment of herpes, HPV, and shingles, and Lauricidin will be included as a recommended part of the protocol. I also advise people that this website (www.natropractica.com) is the only legitimate source of Lauricidin/monolaurin.

Jaquelyn McCandless, MD

I have practically every child I've ever treated on Lauricidin and have recommended it to hundreds of other families over the years. Any substance that can actually affect the body can cause someone somewhere to have a negative reaction. I have rarely seen a negative reaction once I learned to start with smaller amounts and build up, and this would be in the form of extra "stimminess" (a word used to describe the sometimes-agitated behavior of autistic children) which usually subsided with lowering of dose.

Dr. Kenneth R. Koles, PhD

The Hep C patients that I see remain symptom-free and refuse to be tested; herpes sufferers have either completely stopped having outbreaks or have almost completely stopped. Last but not least, the people that use Lauricidin regularly haven't been sick in years.

Jim Neilson, DC

I'm a nutritionally oriented chiropractor in Bend, Oregon. Just wanted to put in a good word for how clinicians like myself are using monolaurin-Lauricidin. I am finding it useful for colds, flus, and yeast overgrowth. I have a couple of people using it for herpes outbreaks. In the natural health field we are always looking for better approaches to these problems. Lauricidin appears to be a new weapon for these problems and an alternative to herbals such as oregano oil and grapefruit seed extract. Lauricidin is also an alternative to other fatty acid products such as caprylic acid from coconut oil and undecenoic acid from castor bean.

Terry Suttles, Nutritional Practitioner

Most people with chronic disease have guts that do not function well, not to mention the liver. Lauricidin is one of the best products I have ever used as an antimicrobial and an immune modulator, and there is some evidence it may help with detoxification. I, a nutritionist, have many clients on it including my 24-year-old daughter who is >80% recovered. I have clients who are terrified to run out of it. It must be used correctly but it is an incredible product.

Charles P. Whalen, DC

I have been recommending Lauricidin to my patients for two years.

I am pleasantly surprised every day by the amazing results that they get from using Lauricidin on a daily basis. Long-term fungal and viral infections disappearing, not getting colds or the flu, stronger immune systems—the list goes on. The anti-fungal, anti-bacterial, and antiviral properties of Lauricidin are helping my patients get and stay healthy. I continue to recommend it to all my friends and patients.

Lay Testimonials
(results for individuals may vary)

HERPES VIRUS

We spoke almost two years ago when herpes outbreaks on my face seemed worsened by the Lauricidin; fortunately the outbreaks decreased when I dropped the dosage and have not returned though I've continued on Lauricidin as prescribed by my physician. Since I've had periodic herpes outbreaks my whole life, this change has been most welcome.

—SONOMA, CA

I ordered six bottles of Lauricidin from you four months ago and would like to order six more. This stuff is amazing. It took about three months to really build up, but I am skipping my Zovirax now regularly and sometimes forget the last time I have taken it. For 15 years that has never happened. I'm really impressed. I did double up on the dose to 6 to 8 scoops a day to get these results, but I couldn't be happier. Please let me know if this dose is safe. I hope so because it's awesome.

—KALISPELL, MT

Dr. Kabara's response: "Safe but maybe not necessary when you reach an outbreak-free condition. Try lowering the amount that still keeps you healthy."

I am a 50-year-old young woman. I've had genital herpes for 30 years. I always have had to take medication for the herpes: first whenever I had an outbreak, then I was having them so often I was put on a lower dose taken daily. I'd miss one dose, and it would start up. I'm telling you this to show you that I've had herpes that have gradually gotten much worse. I know this is not the case with most people. I have found L-lysine to be helpful but for me it still wasn't enough. The good news is that by checking Dr. Weil's site (www.drweil.com) I found my life saver!

It's monolaurin, sold through the researcher Dr. Kabara who developed it (as Lauricidin). I only buy it through Dr. Kabara's site as the price is really good, and I know the quality I'm taking. I hope this doesn't sound like an ad—I just want to share it with all that have this awful problem. I've been taking this for a year. I'm off all medication and have gotten to where I only take the Lauricidin twice a week! I stopped for two weeks, and had a breakout; I wanted to see if it had gone away. (The doctor says that it doesn't but I just had to check.) But still—this is great. I'm going to be posting this on a couple other sites on this forum. It's hard to tell which postings people look at, and I really do want to share it. Good luck.
   —CINCINNATI, OH

I've been using Lauricidin for about two years now and I'm extremely happy with the results. I've had no side effects at all and have not had one outbreak since taking it. Every once in a while when I feel I may be close to an outbreak, I increase my dosage for a couple of days and it goes away.
   —CHATSWORTH, CA

I am a 54-year-old woman and have had major outbreaks of genital herpes since I was 20. I've gone through all the drugs trying to keep it under control but was not too successful. I started Lauricidin about one and a half years ago. The only outbreak I've had was when I was feeling so good I forgot to take it. In fact, I've told everyone I can think of who might benefit. Thank you for this wonderful supplement that has changed my life!

　—GRAND RONDE, OR

I was one of those cases who had constant breakouts with miserable pain. I think I now have the best formula for me. I take two scoops of Lauricidin three times a day and now have no outbreaks (I mean none). I'm extremely grateful for this natural alternative to antivirals.

　—THE VILLAGES, FL

I've had very good results with monolaurin. I have herpes simplex and it has affected my mobility in my neck even when I wasn't having an outbreak. I also struggle with candida overgrowth. I already take a product called "nature's biotic," which helps considerably and decreased my outbreaks as well, but when I added monolaurin I had major life improvement. Warning, start slowly, this is a long-term process and there is a "die-off" effect. You might have a small outbreak, but it clears up quickly. I had great improvement in three weeks. Amazingly, I regained full mobility of my neck. I also had a frozen shoulder from an injury last year and have made remarkable progress in gaining mobility again. I'm able to get back to being more physically active and working out again.

　—LUCY, INTERNET CHAT GROUP

I am taking Monolaurin for herpes. Since I have started taking it, I have not had a breakout, despite being under a lot of stress with the sickness and passing of my mother.

I have been taking the supplement for several months now—twice a day—and I strongly believe it has suppressed my outbreaks of herpes, which were very regular previously.
—TUCSON, AZ

Lauricidin is a wonder—I have not had a cold sore since last September, and I usually get them *at least* once monthly, more often in extreme cold and heat—bad ones, too. I will continue to use it on a daily basis.
—BROOKLYN, NY

I have been feeling better. Outbreak-free for nearly a year. Red marine algae gave me similar results when I first started taking it (back in 1998), but the formulas kept changing and so did the effects. Toward the end of using the RMA it wasn't really doing too much. That is when I did some research and found your product, and it seems to be very helpful for my situation.
—DAYTON, OH

I just wanted to let others know that I have been using Lauricidin for three months and have not had an outbreak of herpes despite being under a great amount of stress and even eating some chocolate and peanuts. I had used valtrex but I would develop a small, painful lesion on some portion of my back a couple of weeks after having had an outbreak. I don't think valtrex was good for me—it suppressed the virus and that's all it did, and I think the virus popped out as that small back lesion. I have not had any symptoms with Lauricidin. This is definitely superior to pharmaceutical antivirals. You can get the website by putting the name "Lauricidin" into a search engine. Good luck.

—INTERNET CHAT GROUP

I've been really ashamed to have contracted this disease, Doctor. The worst part is the emotional consequences and the limited choices for future relationships. I seem to get "purple marks" in various places all over my body ever since I got herpes. I was tested for the very serious K-hsv and don't have that. I never knew there were so many varieties. I was getting a "mosquito-like" bump every few weeks on my thigh, and as long as I take Lauricidin, I don't get the bump and it is rare when I get the purple marks.

—AUSTIN, TX

Hi, I am new to this forum, but not to genital herpes, which I have had since I was a teen and am now 41. I have agonized after being infected. My heart goes out to each and every one of you! Here is the good news I have experienced! I have done a lot of research. I have taken a product called "Lauricidin" for two years and I no longer have any outbreaks. Formerly I would get outbreaks every single month. I prayed that my children would never be infected, and thankfully they were not. I was thinking last night that I need to share this with others. I would not even think of sharing this if I had not been helped one hundred percent. My doctors do not understand it at all! Please go and look up "Lauricidin" on a Web search. It is nontoxic. I pay $30 a jar, and the jar lasts me over a month. It comes in granules. I buy it from the Med-Chem Labs.

Dr. Wilde has talked about it on his site also. I have been on many prescriptions throughout the years but nothing has helped me before—in fact, everything made me feel worse. I am not getting anything out of sharing this except the joy of helping others. Please let me know how it goes!

—UNKNOWN—CUREZONE.COM

FLU/COLDS/SINUSES

My experience with Lauricidin is interesting. My wife and I took it for three to four days. Then we forgot and have been taking it only when we feel a cold or sickness coming on. About a half dozen times we both felt a sickness coming on and we took it [a full scoop] at 6 pm and one at 10 pm, before bed. Every time we woke up with symptoms gone. We went to Las Vegas this last weekend, and after flying on a plane we felt a sore throat and stuffiness coming on— now it too is gone. My wife calls them the magic pebbles.

—WOODSIDE, CA

I want to mention that I think your Lauricidin helped me with the cold/sinus symptoms I wrote you about three weeks ago. And hopefully it has started on my staph epidermidis overgrowth. I've been able to breathe more freely than I have in a very long time since I had two immense sinus clearings a week apart during that cold. The clearings were notable for the quantity and unusually bright yellow color. I've never had anything like that before, and prior to that I'd always had a stuffy nose. I'd just moved up to four scoops daily the week before the cold came on, and it certainly seems like Lauricidin had something to do with it (my recovery).

—NORRISTOWN, PA

For more than four years I've had a chronic sinus condition but no infection of a cold or fever ensuing. My doctor determined that it was a fungal infection because of the greenish stuff. Previously I only used salt-water irrigation. Since I started on Lauricidin, I've been free of phlegm for five and a half months now. If I missed too many days, like when I ran out of the product, my sinus problem would reappear. My sinus is drier and I can speak without constant throat-clearing.

My husband has a chronic allergy-like cough. After reading your website and taking the Lauricidin, he has become a believer. Lauricidin seems to be saving the day! I love it!

—MIAMI SPRINGS, FL

My daughter and I start taking Lauricidin when we feel like we are getting a cold or sinus infection. I am proud to say that I suffered with the sinus problem quiet frequently until I started the Lauricidin. I did not have one the entire year of 2002 and 2003. We were out of Lauricidin just recently and my daughter got a full-blown sinus infection. It really works for us.

—BEAVERCREEK, OH

I have ordered and am currently using Lauricidin, as is my wife and four-year-old child. We have been enjoying a flu- and cold-free winter so far, for the most part. My four-year-old had been taking Lauricidin (eight to ten tablets once or twice a day) for two or three days when he got a slight cold that lasted only two days instead of the normal two to three weeks. He is extremely asthmatic when he gets colds and usually ends up on inhaled steroids and inhaled albuterol for almost a month when he gets any respiratory condition. This time the sick plan was ended after two days of preventative treatments.

—WEATOGUE, CT

Zero flu in this house and not one cold lasting beyond two days. Colin still remains without diarrhea and sleeping through the night, both gains he got from the very start of using Lauricidin. Five months ago we started my seven-year-old son on Lauricidin (two scoops daily). His immediate reaction was change of stool habits, from loose, sometimes explosive stools, to perfect stools overnight. There has been only one bout of diarrhea since, when he was exposed to a pesticide at school. He still remains negative to herpes 1 and 2. EBV remains negative.

—REDFORD, MI

I don't have any baseline/later tests which specifically prove that Lauricidin was solely responsible for any improvements (LYME); I was mixing Lauricidin with other remedies, so cannot extract out exactly what did what. Everything is either empirical or observation. Amongst my friends, whom I've told about Lauricidin, and some of whom are taking it, they report fewer colds; and improvement once a cold begins (shorter duration).

—HONOLULU, HI

I knocked down a rapid-onset cold in two days (sneezing every five to ten minutes and head dripping so bad I couldn't lean over to fill out forms at my PT job with REI last Wednesday eve)! You Rock!

PS—Also small warts are going away (not raised very much, but five to six appeared on my knuckles early this year). They turned bright pink after a week or so, then got dry; now diminished by 50% of original.

—RALEIGH, NC

HEPATITIS C

I haven't tried Lauricidin myself but have seen miraculous results in my wife's and friends' health while taking it. A friend of mine has been coping with hepatitis C, fibromyalgia, and numerous other ailments for almost thirty years. Lately she has been lying around trying to sleep all the time. The pain and fatigue have been unbearable for her—until the other day when she decided the try an experiment. She started taking Lauricidin for the first time. Her husband couldn't believe it: That night she slept the whole night without waking. Since then she has been getting out of bed more, being more active, her pain has eased, and everyone is talking about how much healthier she looks. In my opinion, this is a miracle drug if there ever was one.

—ASHLAND, KENTUCKY

I saw my doctor when I was taking a half scoop of Lauricidin BID. He tested me and upped my dosage to three full scoops a TID. I immediately broke out with a rash, which went away in a few days. I seem to be tolerating about two and a half scoops a day. Bottom line, my Hep PCR qaunt is down and [Lauricidin] is in large part responsible for the ever-increasing drop in my viral load. It's by far the most amazing supplement I've ever been on. I believe I have even dissolved a nuisance fibroid recently, and I attribute it to the Lauricidin, without a doubt.

—SOMERSWORTH, NH

When he first started taking monolaurin eight years ago, his ALT went from 562 to 120 in about two years. This last test was the biggest jump we've seen, from 238 to 469 in six months. These past six months were the only time he *wasn't* using monolaurin. We were trying a different approach with alpha-lipoic acid and selenium. Obviously, this didn't work. Michael has no symptoms at all. He used to deal with fatigue and depression before we stated monolaurin therapy, but that is long gone.

—NORTH AURORA, IL

I have Hep C, contracted through a blood transfusion. It has attacked my liver and caused damage to it also. Been going to several doctors through my HMO providers and couldn't get any relief from them. I then went to my chiropractor because of neuropathy in my feet to see if he could provide any relief. After about six weeks of treatment he told me of an incredible new (at least to me) "dietary supplement." It was Lauricidin. I took the required doses to begin with and now I am taking three scoops a day, two in the morning and one at bedtime. My next visit to the liver doctor indicated through blood tests that not only were my liver assessments actually getting better, there was a complete halt with no new trace of any damage from my Hep C.

I believe this is due to Lauricidin, along with a good diet and vitamins I take daily also. Thank you, Lauricidin, I truly believe that you are playing a major role in my daily health regimen.

—GRANADA HILLS, CA

My girlfriend just got diagnosed with Bell's palsy [a weakness of the nerve that supplies the muscles of the face] recently (Ramsy

Hunt version), and as I am a frequent visitor here [to this website] for Tourette's and OCD, I decided to check your section out.

Virus! That seems to be a common thread here (as it is in Tourette's too) so I wanted to share what my son is taking that is working wonders! It is called Lauricidin, which is a brand name for a lipid called monolaurin. Monolaurin is found in saw palmetto, coconut, and mother's milk! We swear by it. With Tourette's it seems like every little cold or bug going around really acts as a tic trigger, and in fact many believe that the condition is initially triggered by strep or at least exacerbated by it (it was in my son's case). Taking the Lauricidin keeps all that stuff away.

There was a tummy bug going around his class. It only lasted a few days for those who got it, but I was bracing for the worst because I knew if he got it, it would bring him to his knees (tic-wise). He didn't get it. You have to understand—he got *everything* that was going around before taking this. He didn't get it and almost everyone in his class did. I was ecstatic!

Tourette's also can have a yeast overgrowth component, and the Lauricidin has allowed him to go off his Nystatin (internal yeast killer), which has been great. Anyway, I thought I'd share this product with you all in the hopes that you could avoid future outbreaks.

I had shingles twice, and after seeing his amazing results have started taking it too.

—INTERNET CHAT GROUP

CHRONIC FATIGUE/FIBROMYALGIA

I have consumed literally gallons of high-grade coconut oil in the past eighteen months since I read about its supposed healing miracles. Since I am still very ill, I have to say it has done absolutely nothing for my CFIDS/CFS/FMS/neurotoxins/stealth/whatever else you'd like to call this illness. I love the taste of the high-grade oil I purchase online and continue to use it, and extra-virgin olive oil elsewhere in my diet, for that reason only. But as far as anything else goes, I'd put my money on Lauricidin any day. Just five tiny pellets twice daily hit me hard by the third day. I decided to give it a try after reading about it on this list [an Internet site] and started at a very low dose since I'm very reactive and have been ill and disabled for many years. After eleven months I've worked up to just two scoops daily and will continue to slowly titrate upwards.

As for other brands of monolaurin and the Lauricidin brand ... a homeopathic group recently tested me for the efficacy of several monolaurin options, along with whole unsweetened coconut milk. The whole milk turned out to be the most beneficial. It probably won't be practical for me to use though, so I was gratified to hear that Lauricidin came out on top [was the most effective] compared to the other monolaurin brands, for me and also for five other individuals tested at the same time.

—MORRISTOWN, PA

I am so grateful there is a product out there like Lauricidin that could help me get healthy in a safe way. Within a month of using Lauricidin my energy level tripled, and as a result I'm a much happier person.

—JAMAICA PLAIN, MA

I have been using Lauricidin since October 2001. My experience has been very positive with my fatigue issues. I've tried to stop using Lauricidin several times, and my fatigue comes right back. I now continue to use Lauricidin on a daily basis, and it has allowed me to get back to a fairly normal life.

—NOTTINGHAM, PA

The first three days of one scoop twice a day produced an immediate increase in energy lasting all day, along with clearer thinking and deeper, longer sleep. I listened to my body in regard to how much and how often I ingest Lauricidin. The results have been excellent and I am very grateful for this wonderful product.

—SAN ANSELMO, CA

My doctor, who also has fibromyalgia, has me on the supplement Lauricidin. I couldn't live without it. There was one time when I was running low and didn't order in time for it to arrive before I ran out. I was without it for two days. Those were two very painful days, and I learned to make sure I never ran out again.

—INTERNET CHAT GROUP

AUTISM

Michael was diagnosed PDD/NOS (Pervasive Development Disorder/Not Otherwise Specified) at age two in February 2001 by his doctor and referred to an Easter Seals program for integration therapies. It was at age twenty months that Michael developed a severe diaper rash and diarrhea. It was around this time that the symptoms of autism were slowly developing. Michael became moodier, depressed, less manageable. During this time, Michael's stools were runny and his behavior out of control. Tantrums were to the extreme. All previous language lost, no eye contact, no play skills, increased hyperactivity, spinning and increased repetitive behaviors. Toe walking and hand flapping were prominent.

Lauricidin has been nothing short of miraculous in controlling the yeast! Another therapy has been the injection of vitamin B12 shots (0.05mg/ml) two to three times weekly. We noticed longer sentences and an increase in expressive language. As soon as we improved Michael's nutritional status and reduced the gut bugs, we started chelation therapy again and we have seen incredible gains in language, behavior, imaginative play, memory, and social skills. His cheeks and ears no longer turn bright red.

For the first time in two years, Michael's Great Smokes test results came back with 4+ lactobacillus species and 4+ bifidobacteria! I attribute this to the Lauricidin and megadoses of Natren's Mega Dolphilus and Bifido Factor products, as well as three to four capsules of Culturelle daily. His Great Plains lab results are also significantly improved. His arabinose went down from an average of 200 to 58.09 mmol.

The extent of Michael's recovery (two years later) as he approaches his fifth birthday is evidenced today by his many behavioral and intellectual skill improvements. His memory is sharp. He can tell you the name of just about every car on the road, make and model. His interest in model trains has afforded him a wealth of technical details on this subject as well as information about various states across the country. He has an interest in the American Flag and all of our nation's flag songs. He is interested in current comic characters Spiderman and Hulk, preferring books over movies about them. His most recent, amazing personality trait is his sense of humor and ability to tell "knock, knock jokes" and other simple one-line jokes. And most importantly, Michael has genuine, reciprocal relationships with family and peers.

—INTERNET CHAT GROUP

Lauricidin is felt to be more potent than regular capsule monolaurin. My friend noted an improvement and commented today after a trip to Costco about how calm both of our kids were and how with-it my (autistic) son was—opening his own door, climbing in, shutting it, buckling up, and saying earlier, "Oh here, let me help you, Dad" (to carry a package).

—SILVERDALE, WA

I order Lauricidin for my eleven-year-old autistic son, who has been plagued with bacterial, fungal, and viral infections. He now takes two full scoops a day, and without running tests to verify the absence of infection, I believe it has been working well for him. He tolerates it well also. I have taken it myself though not consistently—trying to keep him supplied with all his supplements tends to make me come in second, ah well—I have managed, however, to not get the crud/flu that everyone else in my community seems to have.

—TAHOE CITY, CA

My son, who is now twelve, has really benefited from Lauricidin. He began taking it just over a year ago and continues to take a scoop twice a day. After an initial three-week die-off period, he stabilized at a much healthier level than before. It has not cured him but does seem to be an important part of his overall ongoing treatment for a dysregulated immune system, including a viral overload, by keeping him on more of an even health level as opposed to previous wild swings in health. If he skips a dose, we do notice that he shows more signs of allergy/immune weakness for a few days.

—PIANO, TX

Hi. I just wanted to thank you for your prompt shipment to us this past week. I have a twenty-three-month-old PDD/NOS son who is close to losing his diagnosis due to diet/supplement /enzyme intervention. And the wonderful grace of a loving God. One of the most heart-breaking parts of this disease is when the child cannot reciprocate with affection. I miss my child putting his head on my shoulder for comfort, but there has been a "wall" there now for months. To me it is the most difficult part of this. Tonight he sat in my lap and allowed me to cuddle him without being "stiff" for the first time in months. What a gift and way to start the New Year. I truly believe your product Lauricidin was a big part of this latest improvement.

—AUBURN, AL

I want to share with you some of the changes we have already seen in our son (diagnosed with autism, age eight), which I had at first not attributed to the Lauricidin. I expected changes to come in the area of speech, but instead he has increased focus and shows new interest in books and interactive computer games (sometimes he had only to a very limited degree). He also has been much happier and vocalizing more (he is nonverbal). I have added no new supplements, so it must be this one.

—BUENA PARK, CA

We have just started a product that might be of interest to this thread (the ongoing Internet chat). It is called Lauricidin and is antibacterial, antifungal, and antiviral. We have taken my son off Nystatin, and usually within a week a kind of mental fogginess creeps in—the yeast doing its beastly stuff—but that hasn't happened so far and it's been almost a month, so I believe the product is working. It is made from coconut and is a form of monolaurin—found in mother's milk, saw palmetto, etc. I have been so pleased with the results that I have started to take it for my cold sores that I get quite frequently (gee, I wonder why? could it be all the stress?) with super results too! We chose this route because it was taking care of so much more than the Nystatin alone, and regular Nystatin (liquid) has yellow and red dye in it—not to mention sugars of some sort! We had to get the Nystatin specially compounded, which wasn't so bad but the refrigeration was tough on outings. Anyway, just wanted to share this!

—GISELLE, INTERNET CHAT GROUP

With all of the monolaurin discussion, I thought I would share my daughter's progress on it. She has now been on it for sixteen days. In that time, she has gone from eating only three different foods to trying at least six new ones. She seems to be overcoming texture issues. She also is eating a lot more, so I suspect her gut is healing from something being killed off. The other development has been language increase. She has gone from using words one at a time to name objects, to saying a few two- and three-word phrases. She has also changed her personality and is becoming a little bit mischievous!! When we tested her, her vaccine titers were all high, especially measles, and that is why I decided to try the monolaurin. We still are not all the way up to the dosage Dr. McCandless recommended, so I hope to see more improvement. The only negative reaction we have seen was a rash for a few days, which I assume was die-off, because it seems to have gone away.

—SG, SWITZERLAND

When Cohn's titers were lowered, his EEG was clean. He slept through the night, he remembered what he learned the previous day, his speech improved (receptive and expressive). **The one and only diet change that occurred during this "trial" was the Lauricidin.** He's not cured but has received significant relief, and removing that problem has let us see possibly the bigger problem in him.

—IRVINE, TX

For the past week, we've been using something new, Lauricidin, for tackling yeast. I LOVE the GSE (grapefruit seed extract) but wanted to rotate with something else—in particular something that does not kill good bacteria. Lauricidin does not kill good bacteria, but kills bad bacteria, yeast, and even viruses. Since we've been doing all of these anti-yeast meds and herbals, I started to think that maybe my son's bad bacteria needs to be addressed too. So we started Lauricidin and we have been getting a real good die-off from it—his BMs have a very pathogenic smell to them. If this stuff helps out my son's stubborn yeast, it's got to be good.

—PEORIA, IL

No mixed reviews here. My son started on Lauricidin February 13, 2002. By the next day we had said goodbye to loose stools. By

May we said goodbye to extremely high HHV-6 titers. By September of the same year we had a clean 24-hour EEG. Nothing else was mixed into that biochem equation. He's now nine and his EEG remains clear, his stools and pH normal, and his HHV-6 titers normal. We did not start at a few pellets a day but at a half scoop. We're at one scoop twice a day now . . . for life! The rest of the family takes it, too.

—POSTED ON CSB NOVEMBER 12, 2003

FUNGAL INFECTIONS

I have used Lauricidin as a preventative for flu and have gotten the nice side effect of no longer having toenail fungus. I feel better and have more energy. I think it's an amazing product, and I am grateful to Dr. Kabara for having discovered it, found a way to make it easy to take, and especially for making available at such a low price to the public.

—RENO, NV

I have a history of toenail fungus. I have taken Lamisil in the past but I am a heart patient, so I decided to take Lauricidin orally instead. I have had more results in three months taking Lauricidin than I had in a year taking Lamisil. I am very pleased with my results with Lauricidin, and I intend to continue using these products.

—SPRINGFIELD, MO

I have been a patient of Dr. Whalen for two years now. During the course of treatment, he introduced me to Lauricidin. I had a fungal growth on the back of my ear that did not go away with the drugs and medication prescribed by my family doctor; it just got worse. After taking Lauricidin for two months it is completely gone.

Thank you, Dr. Whalen, for your care and for introducing me to the benefits of Lauricidin.

—REDFORD, MI

MISCELLANEOUS REPORTS

Lauricidin has saved my life! No doubt about it! Last December I was at the end of my rope from illness caused by exposure to toxic molds—my levels of aflatoxins, satratoxins, and trichothecene were causing me to go into *anaphylactic shock* reactions on almost anything I came in contact with, from oranges to deodorant. My "T Killer" cells were at a critically low count.

Last Christmas (2002) I was suicidal because I could not imagine going on any further, and I had no family or financial help for recovery. And due to the mold I had already lost my home, my job, and I had no way out.

I was taking major dosages of the Lauricidin from day one. Then the incredible thing was that within about 3 days I had this *major energy spurt* and felt like a normal person again! Something was working!

I couldn't believe it! I could get out of bed, and I felt like "doing" something. This was short-lived, but it was better than anything that had happened in more than a year.

I now have been on the Lauricidin for over a year and am not backing off the dosage I am taking. In fact, when I am under major stress or may have been exposed to some virus, I up the dosage for a few days.

Recognized Improvements:

Documented tests that Killer Cells are being restored to normal, healthier levels.

Documented nutritional balances are being restored.

Brain/thought patterns are being restored—can work and process mentally (work extensively on computer, write, read, teach, and hold a conversation).

Neurological damage is diminishing.

Digestive system can process foods now.

Have a much healthier appearance: healthy skin and hair; liver spots disappearing.

Pocks (holes) in skin are regenerating.

Have ENERGY!! Can function for twelve to fourteen hours a day now! Working a job again.

I'm sure there is more I could include because my whole body has been affected, but this gives a general picture of recovery. I do know for myself that I am now finally recovering from the mold exposure, and I have *hope* of my having "life" again.

I thank God and Dr. Kabara for the wonderful supplement that has been put in my hands. It works!

—WHITEWATER, KS

I originally started using Lauricidin for my cat's herpes to the eye, but I ended up using it more for myself and my family than the cat. It has helped my father with his prostate cancer, my mother with her intestinal problems, and myself with a severe sinus problem I've had for years. What a difference Lauricidin has made in my life!

—ALPHARETTA, GA

A voice from England: Saturday I met Bernard and Rowena Halle, each of whom give you every credit for Bernard's much increased quality of life. After being chair-bound with cancer for four years, he is up and about, filled with enthusiasm and has just finished cleaning out his barn, building a workshop, and pursuing his hobby—making furniture.

—UNITED KINGDOM

I just wanted to submit my very grateful testimony for (so far!) benefits. I caught a fungal infection in my hairline and all over my scalp that left me for three years with falling out hair, balding patches, red itchy bumps, and really gross scaly nonstop peeling dandruff-y conditions inside the hairline. Disgusting! I tried everything the doctors gave me: antifungal pills, some costing as much as $150 a bottle, shampoos, you name it. Then my alternatively minded doctor got me a container of your Lauricidin, and within a week of taking it religiously I was brushing my hair one day and noticed that my scalp looked clear! It's still clear, and I've been off the Lauricidin, for a few weeks (ran out!). Still clear! Thank you so much for your wonderful product! I am a very pretty woman in my early thirties, and it was really debilitating to worry about that gross, nasty, fungal scalp thing constantly!

—MALIBU, CA

Just wanted to drop you a line to say "Thanks!" I've suffered with acne since I was about ten (I'm now twenty-four). A few years ago I was put on antibiotics for my skin and they did a great job of clearing it up. I was on them for four to five years, and my skin was practically flawless. Then I moved and had to get a new derma-

182

tologist. When she saw what medications I was on for my skin, she couldn't stop laughing. She said, "Who prescribed this to you? No one prescribes these anymore! They can totally screw up your liver." Well, without the antibiotics my skin got so bad that I was crying almost every day. I had cysts all over my face that would not go away and hurt. It was the pain that really got me. The doctor wouldn't refill my prescription, and the topicals she gave me made my skin even worse. I did some research, and at acne.org I found definitions of different kinds of acne. One of them was a bacterial infection that can happen after prolonged use of antibiotics; because I had never had acne this bad until I came off the antibiotics it seemed a reasonable culprit.

One day while on the Internet, looking up something unrelated, I came across the site for Lauricidin. The site didn't claim any results with acne, but the antibiotic properties of Lauricidin made me think it might work. After emailing Dr. K and looking at the site for a few days I decided it would be worth a try. He said it could take a few months for anything to happen. But after taking Lauricidin for two or three days new cysts stopped forming, and after those went away no more new ones came back! So now I just take Lauricidin and use benzoyl peroxide topically, and I don't have any more outbreaks—only a stray pimple with my period. It's amazing ... I have to say I didn't expect it to work, but it did and I thank God and you. Thank you!

—BIRMINGHAM, AL

I've been meaning to write to you regarding Lauricidin. I'm not sure of the studies you've done with this product, but I want you to know how it's helped me. I have dealt with colitis for the last five years. I used a Rowasa medication two to three times a week to keep it under control. About three weeks after starting to take your product I noticed that I wasn't having flare-ups as regularly and now not at all. I haven't had to use my medication in over a month and am so very happy about it. I have to believe that it is this product making the difference. I'm only on my second jar and already feeling great.

—GALENA, IL

I have suffered from herpes, which generally erupts when I eat chocolate (I'm a chocolate addict and find it very hard to give up). Herpes can be very distressing emotionally, and I'm determined to beat it. Lauricidin does not work straight away, but at present I am getting no outbreaks although I have only been taking it for two months. I have a twelve-month supply and will let you know if I get any more outbreaks over this period.

The positive side of suffering with herpes is that it makes you realize just how sensitive your body is. For example, stress, sugar, and chocolate often cause me instant tingling sensations, which is an indication that the virus is reactivating. I have also noticed when taking Lauricidin that the tingling goes away, and since I now take it every day I hope I will never suffer another outbreak. For me it seems like a reasonable investment.

It's impossible for me to know how well Lauricidin really works, but time will tell. All I can say is that formerly if I ate a box of Jaffa Cakes this would result in instant outbreaks, but now nothing happens so I am hopeful.

The most depressing aspect of suffering viruses and other illnesses is that we all want a cure, and some people take advantage of this need by lying or claiming they have found a cure. For some reason I felt that Lauricidin seemed to be genuine and the website very professional. It has also been approved [as a food supplement] by the FDA.

Another interesting fact is that my brother has suffered quite a nasty cold lately, and yesterday I did sneeze a couple of times but today I have no symptoms. Meanwhile my brother looks shattered, so maybe Lauricidin has other benefits.

I found out that I was HIV positive in February of 2004 and had tests done every two months until February of 2005, after which I started a schedule of testing every three months. Toward the end of 2005 I began taking 400 µg of selenium and 1 scoop of Lauricidin (which is three grams of monolaurin) daily.

Below is a "chart" of my test results.

04-Feb	CD4 390	viral load	2377 copies/ml.
04-April	CD4 560	viral load	591 copies/ml.
04-June	CD4 528	viral load	591 copies/ml.
04-Aug	CD4 675	viral load	7684 copies/ml.
04-Oct	CD4 729	viral load	2474 copies/ml.
04-Dec	CD4 800	viral load	1780 copies/ml.
05-Feb	CD4 702	viral load	237 copies/ml.
05-May	CD4 303	viral load	1260 copies/ml.
05-Aug	CD4 242	viral load	950 copies/ml.
05-Oct	CD4 238	viral load	1830 copies/ml.

Started taking Lauricidin—one scoop (~2.8 grams) 05-Dec

06-Jan	CD4 213	viral load	1790 copies/ml.
06-Apr	CD4 263	viral load	1150 copies/ml.
06-Jul	CD4 257	viral load	557 copies/ml.
06-Oct	CD4 250	viral load	628 copies/ml.
06-Nov	CD4 250	viral load	600 copies/ml.

As you can see, aside from some fluctuation (which is to be expected), I have seen nothing but improvement overall, and I am really excited about the VL count from this last test. The numbers are so close to that magic "undetectable" mark. Let me mention that I'm not on any HIV meds.

—THAILAND

We are a regular customer of Lauricidin, and a very happy one at that. Lauricidin has been a key to helping my daughter overcome alopecia hair loss . . .

—YORK, ME

Prevention of Dental Caries by Monolaurin

See the Reference lists in the back of the book for sources that give a complete account of fatty acids and their ester forms as antimicrobial agents. The following table demonstrates monolaurin's high activity against gram-positive strains of bacteria. It was not active against gram-negative organisms.

In Vitro Studies with Lauricidin

TABLE 13.1

Effect of pH on MIC Values (ppm) of Lauricidin

Organism	pH			
	5.0	**6.0**	**7.0**	**8.0**
Gram-negative				
Escherichia coli	>1000	>1000	>1000	>1000
Ps aeruginosa	500	>1000	>1000	>1000
Gram-positive				
Staphylococcus aureus	NG	62.5	250	125
Streptococcus agalactiae	15.6	15.6	15.6	15.6
Streptococcus mutans	15.6	15.6	31.2	15.6
Streptococcus sanguis	15.6	31.2	31.2	31.2

NG = no growth

Streptococcal organisms are more susceptible to inhibition by Lauricidin than are *Staphylococcal* organisms. The activity of Lauricidin was only somewhat affected by pH. There was no difference in MIC values among different strains of the same species, or different species of the same genus, as demonstrated by values for *Streptococcal* organisms.

Test tube data on the inhibitory activity of monolaurin was obtained on *Streptococcus mutans*. This organism is the most important etiological agent for producing dental caries. Growth or inhibition was monitored by following changes in population number as a function of time. With a starting concentration of approximately 500,000 colony-forming units of *S. mutans*, Lauricidin at a concentration of 32 ppm or less inhibited growth.

In Vivo Results Using Lauricidin

It is widely accepted that growth and metabolic products of microorganisms are chiefly responsible for tooth decay. An antibacterial agent shown to be active in a test tube cannot be assumed effective in the body. Our research group conducted experiments using a rat caries model. The model initially chosen by the Michigan State University food science group led by Dr. Schemmel was adopted from the National Institute of Dental Research (NIDR). Rats were weaned at 18 or 20 days of age onto a modified high-sucrose NIH (National Institutes of Health) cariogenic diet. Since 1978 this diet is a readily recognized model for investigating dental caries. Animals were inoculated orally with a standardized bacterial culture at 18–20 days of age. The rats initially were given 50% sucrose water with a standardized microbial culture. After 48 hours, drinking water was changed to pure distilled and given ad libitum (i.e., rats were allowed to choose the amount of food/water on their own) for the duration of the experiment. The experimental groups were placed on diets containing 2% Lauricidin or 2% Crisco.

At the end of the experimental feedings, molar teeth from the lower and upper jaws were evaluated for both microorganisms and caries. In earlier trials, animals on the experimental diets were killed after two, four, and six weeks. Upon examination after two weeks, the microflora population was found to be similar in both control (Crisco) and Lauricidin groups. However, at the four- and six-week intervals, there was a significant decrease (p = 0.05) in total caries and S. mutans in animals receiving 2% Lauricidin. These results were highly significant since they show that an antimicrobial agent in a cariogenic diet lowers the number of organisms that lead to lower dental carie scores.

Our results using Lauricidin were confirmed by Williams et al. (1982). In this study, weanling rats were given high-sucrose cariogenic diets containing 2% lauric acid, linoleic acid, nonanoic acid, or Lauricidin. Plaque accumulation was determined at the conclusion of a 21-day test period. No significant differences were observed among the test groups in food consumption, nor were there any differences in body weight gain. The least amount of plaque was recorded in the animals given monolaurin (Lauricidin); the other fatty acids exerted no significant effect upon plaque accumulation. The dental caries data indicated that the least number of lesions occurred in the animals on the diet containing monolaurin (Lauricidin).

Since the effects noted for dental carie scores were lower than the reduction in bacterial numbers alone, a mechanism other than antimicrobial action of Lauricidin was suggested. Caries formation is the result of cariogenicity induced by the presence of *Streptococcus mutans.* In this animal model system caries are associated with the formation of an adherent and water-insoluble glucan. This glucose plaque polymer, dextran, is formed by the action of an enzyme called glucosyltransferase (GT) on glucose. To test whether or not another mechanism besides antibacterial action was involved in lowering the dental carie scores, GT activity was studied in the presence of the surfactants Lauricidin, sodium lauryl sulfate (SLS), and Tween 80. Lauricidin reduced the total GT enzyme activity 89% to 90% of the control value. SLS was less active, and Tween 80 increased enzyme activity.

These studies indicated that Lauricidin's prevention of dental caries was not only due to its antibiotic effects but also to its effect on the enzyme GT that builds plaque from sugars.

Improved dental health involves a better understanding of how specific proteins and specific fats can influence and neutralize the cariogenic potential of sugars. The research of my team (see references by Kabara et al.) over the past four decades has given us a unique lipid, Lauricidin, which has high *in vivo* cariostatic activity and a nontoxic Generally Regarded As Safe (GRAS) food additive rating. (This rating is only given to additives allowed in food products.) The use of Lauricidin as a dental control agent, therefore, may have as much or more impact on dental caries as fluoride, as it can be easily and safely added to foods as well as dental hygiene products.

Put into a chewing gum, this special lipid (monolaurin) was the subject of a patent (number 4,952,407, assigned to the Wm. Wrigley, Jr., Company) to reduce and remove dental plaque in humans. Lauricidin was shown to be a good dental adjunct for dogs by helping reduce their plaque and bad breath as well.

References

A) Selected References from the Author's Own Bibliography (in chronological order)

Plotz, E. J., J. J. Kabara, M. E. Davis, G. V. LeRoy, and R. G. Gould. 1968. Studies on the synthesis of cholesterol in the brain of a human fetus. *Am J Obstet Gynecol* 101:534–538.

Kabara, J. J., B. B. Chapman, and B. M. Borin. 1972. Effect of hypocholesteremic drugs on tumor-bearing mice. *Proc Soc Exp Biol and Med* 139 (1):100–104.

Kabara, J. J., D. M. Swieczkowski, A. J. Conley, and J. P. Truant. 1972. Fatty acids and derivatives as antimicrobial agents. *Antimicrobial Agents and Chemotherapy* 2 (1): 23–28.

Kabara, J. J., A. J. Conley, D. M. Swieczkowski, I. A. Ismail, Lie Ken Jie, and F. D. Gunstone. 1973. Antimicrobial action of isomeric fatty acids on group A streptococcus. *J Med Chem* 16:1060–1063.

Conley, A. J., and J. J. Kabara. Antimicrobial action of esters of polyhydric alcohols. *Antimicrobial Agents and Chemotherapy* 4:501–506.

Kabara, J. J. Mode of action of antibiotics on microbial walls and membranes. 1974. M. R. J. Salton and A. Tomasy, eds. *Annals of the New York Academy of Sciences* 235:103.

Kabara, J. J., and A. J. Conley. 1974. A non-caloric role for MCT and other lipids, in *Mittelkettige Triglyceride (MCT)*, ed. H. Kaunitz, K. Lang, and W. Fekl, special issue, *Der Diat Zur Zeitschrih Fur Ernahrungswissenschah Supplenta* (17):17–26.

Kabara, J. J. 1975. Lipids as safe and effective antimicrobial agents for cosmetics and pharmaceuticals. *Cosmetics and Perfumery* 90:21–25.

Kabara, J. J., and G. Van Haitsma. 1975. Aminimides II: Antimicrobial effects of short-chain fatty acid derivatives. *JAOCS* 52 (9):444–447.

Kabara, J. J. 1977. Monolaurin as an antimicrobial agent. US Patent 4,002,775, filed n.d., and issued Jan. 1977.

Kabara, J. J., R. Vrable, and M. S. F. Lie Ken Jie. 1977. Antimicrobial lipids: Natural and synthetic fatty acids and monoglycerides. *Lipids* 12:753–759.

Kabara, J. J. 1977. Effect of dietary fat on drug metabolism, in Proceedings of the 13th World Congress Symposium, special issue, *International Society for Fat Research* 3:53–61.

Kabara, J. J. 1977. Skin lipids as antimicrobial substances, in Proceedings of the 13th World Congress Symposium, special issue, *International Society for Fat Research* 3:45–53.

Kabara, J. J. 1978. Synergistic microbiocidal composition and method. US Patent 4,067,997, filed n.d., and issued Jan. 10, 1978.

Preissler, C. J., R. Schemmel, and J. J. Kabara. 1978. Inhibition of *Streptococcus mutans* and dental caries in rats fed carcinogenic diets. *Nutritional Rep Int* 18:27–33.

Kabara, J. J. 1979. Fatty acids and derivatives as antimicrobial agents—A review. In *The Pharmacological Effects of Lipids,* ed. J. J. Kabara, 1–14. Champaign, IL: The American Oil Chemists' Society.

Kabara, J. J., P. Lynch, K. Krohn, and R. Schemmel. 1979. The anti-cariogenic activity of a food-grade lipid—Lauricidin R. In *The Pharmacological Effects of Lipids,* ed. J. J. Kabara, 25–36. Champaign, IL: The American Oil Chemists' Society.

Schemmel, R. A., P. Lynch, K. Krohn, and J. J. Kabara. 1979. Monolaurin as an anticaries agent. In *The Pharmacological Effects of Lipids,* ed. J. J. Kabara, 37–44. Champaign, IL: The American Oil Chemists' Society.

Li, C. Y., and J. J. Kabara. 1979. Effects of Lauricidin on Fomes annosus and Phellinus weirii. In *The Pharmacological Effects of Lipids,* ed. J. J. Kabara, 45–50. Champaign, IL: The American Oil Chemists' Society.

Kabara, J. J. Multi-functional food-grade preservatives in cosmetics. *Drug and Cosmetic Industry* 125:60/76–140/145.

Kabara, J. J. Toxicological, bactericidal and fungicidal properties of fatty acids and some derivatives. *JAOCS* 56:760–767.

Kabara, J. J., ed. 1979. *The Pharmacological Effects of Lipids.* Champaign, IL: The American Oil Chemists' Society.

Kabara, J. J. 1980. GRAS antimicrobial agents for cosmetic products. *J Soc Cosmet Chem* 31:1–10.

Kabara, J. J. 1980. Lipids as host resistance factors of human milk. *Nutrition Reviews* 38:65–73.

Lynch, P., J. J. Kabara, and R. Schemmel. 1980. *Streptococcus mutans* colony forming units and severity of dental caries in rats fed three types of diets with and without Lauricidin. *Microbios Letters* 12:7–13.

Kabara, J. J. 1980. Antimicrobial compositions. US Patent 4,189,481, filed n.d., and issued Feb. 19, 1980.

Kabara, J. J. 1981. The medium is the preservative. *Cosmetics & Toiletries* 96:63–67.

Kabara, J. J. 1981. The changing world and unchanging management. *Cosmetic Technology,* 10–11.

Kabara, J. J. 1981. Food-grade chemicals for use in designing food preservative systems. *J Food Prot* 44:633–657.

Kimsey, H. R., D. M. Adams, and J. J. Kabara. 1981. Increased inactivation of bacterial sporea at high temperatures in the presence of monoglycerides. *J Food Safety* 3:69–82.

Chipley, J. R., L. D. Story, P. T. Todd, and J. J. Kabara. 1981. Inhibition of aspergillus growth and extracellular aflatoxin accumulation by sorbic acid and derivatives of fatty acids. *J Food Safety* 3:109–119.

Nickerson, K. W., V. C. Kramer, and J. J. Kabara. 1982. The effectiveness of Lauricidin preservative systems against detergent-resistant Enterobactercloacae. *Soap/Cosmetics/Chemical Specialties* 58 (2):50–53.

Wernette, C. M., C. L. San Clemente, and J. J. Kabara. 1982. The effects of surfactants upon the activity and distribution of glucosyltransferase in *Streptococcus mutans* 6715. *Pharm & Therap in Dent* 6:99–7.

Schemmel, R. A., K. Krohn-Lutz, P. Lynch, and J. J. Kabara. 1982. Influence of dietary disaccarides on mouth microorganisms and experimental dental caries in rats. *Arch Oral Biol* 27:435–441.

Hierholzer, J. C., and J. J. Kabara. 1982. In vitro effects of monolaurin compounds on enveloped RNA and DNA viruses. *Journal of Food Safety* 4:1–12.

Kabara, J. J. 1982. A new preservative system for food. *Journal of Food Safety* 4:13–34.

Kenney, Dolores with J. J. Kabara. 1982. Cosmetic formulas preserved with food-grade chemicals—Part I. *Cosmetics and Toiletries* 97:71–76.

Kabara, J. J., and C. M. Wernette. 1982. Cosmetic formulas preserved with food-grade chemicals—Part II. *Cosmetics and Toiletries* 97:77–84.

Kabara, J. J. 1982. Dietary lipids as anticariogenic agents, in *Foods, Nutri-*

tion, and Dental Health, eds. J. J. Hefferren and H. M. Koehler, special issue, *American Dental Association* 2:67–96.

Kabara, J. J. 1983. Medium-chain fatty acids and esters. In *Antimicrobials in Foods,* eds. A. L. Brennen and P. M. Davidson, 109–140. New York: Marcel Dekker.

Lynch, P., R. A. Schemmel, and J. J. Kabara. 1983. Anticariogenicity of dietary glycerol monolaurin in rats. *Caries Res* 17:131–138.

Kabara, J. J. 1984. Antimicrobial agents derived from fatty acids. *J American Oil Chemists' Society* 61:397–403.

Kabara, J. J. 1984. Polyene: Nutzen oder schaden? Trans. Ermuthe Idris, MD. *Selecta* 6:414–418.

Kabara, J. J. 1984. Inhibition of *Staphylococcus aureus* in a model agar-meat system by monolaurin: A research note. *J Food Safety* 6:197–201.

Kabara, J. J. 1984. Arteriosklerose—Das risiko der behandlung von risiko-faktosen. *Bulletin of the European Organization for the Control of Circulatory Diseases* 8:57–77.

Kabara, J. J., ed. 1984. *Cosmetic and Drug Preservation: Principles and Practice.* New York: Marcel Dekker.

Kabara, J. J. 1984. Cosmetic preservation: The problems and the solutions. In *Cosmetic and Drug Preservation: Principles and Practice,* ed. J. J. Kabara, 3–6. New York: Marcel Dekker.

Kabara, J. J. 1984. Composition and structure of microorganisms. In *Cosmetic and Drug Preservation: Principles and Practice,* ed. J. J. Kabara, 21–27. New York: Marcel Dekker.

Kabara, J. J. 1984. Medium-chain fatty acids and esters as antimicrobial agents. In *Cosmetic and Drug Preservation: Principles and Practice,* ed. J. J. Kabara, 275–304. New York: Marcel Dekker.

Kabara, J. J. 1984. Lauricidin: The nonionic emulsifier with antimicrobial properties. In *Cosmetic and Drug Preservation: Principles and Practice,* ed. J. J. Kabara, 305–322. New York: Marcel Dekker.

Kabara, J. J. 1984. Food-grade chemicals in a systems approach to cosmetic preservation. In *Cosmetic and Drug Preservation: Principles and Practice,* ed. J. J. Kabara, 339–356. New York: Marcel Dekker.

Schemmel, R. A., and J. J. Kabara. 1985. Fatty acids, monoglycerides and sucrose esters and anticaries agents review. In *The Pharmacologi-*

cal Effects of Lipids II, ed. J. J. Kabara, 51–59. Champaign, IL: American Oil Chemists' Society.

Fletcher, R. D., A. C. Albers, J. N. Albertson, Jr., and J. J. Kabara. 1985. Effect of monoglycerides on mycoplasma pneumoniae growth. In *The Pharmacological Effects of Lipids II,* ed. J. J. Kabara, 59–63. Champaign, IL: American Oil Chemists' Society.

Kabara, J. J. 1985. Inhibition of *Staphylococcus aureus* in a model sausage system by monoglycerides. In *The Pharmacological Effects of Lipids II,* ed. J. J. Kabara, 71–75. Champaign, IL: American Oil Chemists' Society.

Chipley, J. R., P. T. Todd, F. Atchley, and J. J. Kabara. 1985. Effects of fatty acid derivatives on the release of extracellular enzymes from bacteria. In *The Pharmacological Effects of Lipids II,* ed. J. J. Kabara, 97–102. Champaign, IL: American Oil Chemists' Society.

Kabara, J. J., M. Ohkawa, T. Ikekawa, T. Katori, and Y. Nishikawa. 1985. Examinations on antitumor immunological and plant-growth inhibitory effects of monoglycerides of caprylic, capric, and lauric acids and related compounds. In *The Pharmacological Effects of Lipids II,* ed. J. J. Kabara, 263–272. Champaign, IL: American Oil Chemists' Society.

Kabara, J. J., ed. 1985. *The Pharmacological Effects of Lipids II.* Champaign, IL: American Oil Chemists' Society.

Flournoy, D. J., and J. J. Kabara. 1985. The role of Lauricidin as an antimicrobial agent. *Drugs of Today* 21 (8): 373–377.

Kabara, J. J. 1983. Antimicrobial composition for non-medical use consisting mainly of diluted aqueous solution or diluted suspension of palmitoleic acid. Japanese Patent application no. 7405/74. Registration no. 1179254, filed n.d., and issued Nov. 30, 1983.

Kabara, J. J. 1986. Dietary lipids as anticariogenic agents. *Journal of Environmental Pathology, Toxicology and Oncology* 6 (3/4): 87–114.

Kabara, J. J., and George H. Scherr, eds. 1986. *Advances in Human Nutrition,* vol. 3. Park Forest, IL: Chem-Orbital.

Kabara, J. J. 1986. Dietary lipids as cariogenic agents. In *Advances in Human Nutrition,* vol. 3, eds. J. J. Kabara and George H. Scherr, 87–114. Park Forest, IL: Chem-Orbital.

Kabara, J. J., and Mary Beth Brady. 1986. Combination emulsifier/ acidulant extends cheese sauce shelf-life. *Food Processing,* 38–40.

Kabara, J. J. 1987. Fatty acids and esters as antimicrobial/insecticidal agents. In *Ecology and metabolism of plant lipids,* eds. Glenn Fuller and W. David Nes, 220–238. Washington, DC: American Oil Chemists' Society.

Isaacs C.E., Thormar H. 1991. The role of milk-derived antimicrobial lipids as antiviral and antibacterial agents. *Adv. Exp. Med. Biol.* 310: 159–65.

B) Volumes Representing Scholarly Summaries on the Beneficial Effects of Saturated Fats

The following references are for the chapters of *The Pharmacological Effects of Lipids,* Volumes I–III:

Kabara, J. J., ed. 1978. *The Pharmacological Effects of Lipids I.* Champaign, IL: American Oil Chemists' Society.

Kabara, J. J. Fatty acids and derivatives as antimicrobial agents—A review. In Kabara 1978, chapter 1.

Shibasaki, Isao, and Nobuyuki Kato. Combined effects on antibacterial activity of fatty acids and their esters against gram-negative bacteria. In Kabara 1978, chapter 2.

Kabara, J. J., P. Lynch, K. Krohn, and R. Schemmel. The anti-cariogenic activity of a food-grade lipid Lauricidin. In Kabara 1978, chapter 3.

Schemmel, R., P. Lynch, K. Krohn, and J. J. Kabara. Monolaurin as an anticaries agent. In Kabara 1978, chapter 4.

Li, C. Y., and J. J. Kabara. Effects of Lauricidin on *Fomes annosus* and *Phellinus weirii.* In Kabara 1978, chapter 5.

Gershon, Herman, and Larry Shanks. Antifungal activity of fatty acids and derivatives: Structure activity relationships. In Kabara 1978, chapter 6.

Snipes, Wallace, and Alec Keith. Hydrophobic alcohols and di-tert-butyl phenols as antiviral agents. In Kabara 1978, chapter 7.

Sands, Jeffrey A., David D. Auperin, Peter D. Landin, Albert Reinhardt, and Stephen P. Cadden. Antiviral effects of fatty acids and derivatives: Lipid-containing bacteriophages as a model system. In Kabara 1978, chapter 8.

McFarlane, J. E. Fatty acids and insect growth. In Kabara 1978, chapter 9.

Puritch, George S. Biocidal effects of fatty acid salts on various forest insect pests. In Kabara 1978, chapter 10.

Ikeshaji, Toshiaki. Lipids self-limiting the populations of mosquito larvae. In Kabara 1978, chapter 11.

Freese, Ernst. Mechanism of growth inhibition by lipophilic acids. In Kabara 1978, chapter 12.

Mandava, N., and G. R. Chandra. Glucolipids of rape *(Brassica napus L.)* pollen. In Kabara 1978, chapter 13.

Davis, Brian K., Inhibition of fertilizing capacity in mammalian spermatozoa by natural and synthetic vesicles. In Kabara 1978, chapter 14.

Schneider, F. Howard, and Tom Lloyd. Effects of sodium butyrate on mouse neuroblastoma cells in culture. In Kabara 1978, chapter 15.

Tweedle, C. D., and J. J. Kabara. Evidence for a lipophilic nerve sprouting factor(s). In Kabara 1978, chapter 16.

Mickel, Hubert S., Peroxidized arachidonic acid effects on human platelets and its proposed role in the induction of damage to white matter. In Kabara 1978, chapter 17.

Verdonk, G., A. Christophe, R. Mortelmans, and D. T. Andevivere. Possibilities of semi-synthetic fats for human nutrition and dietetics: New concepts in the physio-pathology of lipid assimilation. In Kabara 1978, chapter 18.

Kaunitz, Hans. Toxic effects of polyunsaturated vegetable oils. In Kabara 1978, chapter 19.

Kabara, J. J., ed. 1985. *The Pharmacological Effects of Lipids II.* **Champaign, IL: American Oil Chemists' Society.**

Lands, William E. M. Influence of bond location on the effectiveness of acyl chains. In Kabara 1985, chapter 1.

Adams, Dorothy A., Sara J. Freauff, and Kent L. Erickson. Biophysical characterization of dietary lipid influences on lymphocytes. In Kabara 1985, chapter 2.

Zakim, David, and Yehosua Hochman. Microsomal UDP-glucuronyltransferase as a probe of its lipid environment. In Kabara 1985, chapter 3.

Wisnieski, Bernadine J., and Leora S. Zalman. Photolabeling from inside the membrane reveals factors affecting protein insertion. In Kabara 1985, chapter 4.

Bramhall, John. Permeation of amphiphilic solutes across lipid bilayers. In Kabara 1985, chapter 5.

Schemmel, R., and J. J. Kabara. Fatty acids, monoglycerides and sucrose esters as anticaries agents: A review. In Kabara 1985, chapter 6.

Fletcher, Ronald D., Ann C. Albers, John N. Albertson, Jr., and J. J. Kabara. Effect of monoglycerides on mycoplasma pneumoniae growth. In Kabara 1985, chapter 7.

Baker, Robert C., Winnie Poon, Donna Kline, and Dharma V. Vadehra. Antimicrobial properties of Lauricidin in mechanically deboned chicken, minced fish and chicken sausage. In Kabara 1985, chapter 8.

Kabara, J. J. Inhibition of *Staphylococcus aureus* in a model sausage system by monoglycerides. In Kabara 1985, chapter 9.

Vadehruand, D. V., and V. Wahi. Comparison of antibacterial properties of monolaurin and BHA against antibiotic-resistant and sensitive strains of *Staphylococcus aureus* and *Pseudomonas aeruginosa*. In Kabara 1985, chapter 10.

Vadehra, D. V., V. Wahi, J. Keswani, and P. J. Asnani. Neutralization of antibacterial properties of monolaurin and BHA by tweens. In Kabara 1985, chapter 11.

Chipley, J. R., P. T. Todd, F. Atchley, and J. J. Kabara. Effects of fatty acid derivatives on the release of extracellular enzymes from bacteria. In Kabara 1985, chapter 12.

Kapral, Frank A., and Joel E. Mortensen. The inactivation of bactericidal fatty acids by an enzyme of *Staphylococcus aureus*. In Kabara 1985, chapter 13.

Leisman, Gary B., Michael A. Recny, John S. White, and Lowell P. Hager III. Amphiphilic and proteolytic activivation of *E. coli* pyruvate disease. In Kabara 1985, chapter 14.

Mara, M., J. Julak, Z. Mikova, and C. Michalec. The significance of lipids of scotochromogenic mycobacteria for their identification, taxonomy and immuno-stimulating properties. In Kabara 1985, chapter 15.

Manzoli, Francesco A., Nadir M. Maraldi, and Silvano Capitani. Effect of phospholipids on the control of nuclear DNA template restriction. In Kabara 1985, chapter 16.

Tuhackova, Zdena, and Jan Hradec. The mode of action of cholesteryl 14-methylhexadecanoate in protein synthesis. In Kabara 1985, chapter 17.

Ammon, Helmut V. Effects of fatty acids on intestinal transport. In Kabara 1985, chapter 18.

Oron, Yoram, Etta Nadler, and Monica Lupu. The subcellular site of the cholinergic breakdown of phosphatidylinositol: Implications on the mechanism of calcium influx in the parotid. In Kabara 1985, chapter 19.

Nenzil, Eugene, Jeanne Fourche, and Helene Jensen. Investigations on lipid associations using myelin tube formation. In Kabara 1985, chapter 20.

Mickel, Huber S. Biological effects of lipid peroxides: Lipid peroxidation hypothesis of the etiology of multiple sclerosis. In Kabara 1985, chapter 21.

Sherratt, H. S. A., K. Barlett, and D. M. Turnbull. Four hypoglycaemic compounds that inhibit B-oxidation: 2[5(4-chlorophenyl)pentyl] oxirane-2-carboxyiate (POCA), hypoglycin, pent-4-enoate and valproate: A comparison of their mechanisms of action. In Kabara 1985, chapter 22.

Kabara, J. J., Masanori Ohkawa, Tetsuro Ikekawa, Talsuhiko Kari, and Yoshihiro Nishikawa. Examinations on antitumor, immunological, and plant-growth inhibitory effects of monoglycerides of caprylic, capric, and lauric acids and related compounds. In Kabara 1985, chapter 23.

Berdel, Wolfgang E., Ulrich Fink, Michael Fromm, Bernd Egger, Anneliese Reicherl, Kurl S. Zanker, and Johann Rasteller. Antitumor and antileukemic properties of synthetic alkyl-lysophospholipids (ALP) in vitro. In Kabara 1985, chapter 24.

Berdel, Wolfgang E., Ulrich Fink, Gaby Weiss, Hans P. Emslander, Ingeborg Wust, Jack Nisenhaum, Ekkehard Thiel, Rudolf Babic, Wolfgang Gossner, Johann Rasleller, and Hans Bloemer. Final report on a combined intravenous/oral phase I pilot study of the alkyl-lysophospholipid derivative ET-18-OCH3. In Kabara 1985, chapter 25.

Chang, M. L. W., and M. A. Johnson. Effect of dietary lecithin on lipid metabolism in rats. In Kabara 1985, chapter 26.

Goh, Edward H. Regulation of hepatic cholesterogenesis by exogenous cholesterol investigated with 3H-desmosterol tracer. In Kabara 1985, chapter 27.

Chung, Okkyung Kim, and Yeshajahu Pomeranz. Recent trends in usage of fats and oils as functional ingredients in the baking industry—Nutritive value. In Kabara 1985, chapter 28.

Kabara, J. J., ed. 1989. *The Pharmacological Effects of Lipids III.* **Champaign, IL: American Oil Chemists' Society.**

Farber, Emmanuel. The development of cancer with chemicals—a multistep process. In Kabara 1989, chapter 1.

Lipkin, George, Martin Rosenberg, and Edward Fass. Can modulation of the malignant phenotype by an endogenous inhibitor lead to tumor regression in vivo? In Kabara 1989, chapter 2.

LeRoith, Derek. Evolutionary origins of hormones and tissue growth factors: Possible applications to oncology. In Kabara 1989, chapter 3.

Svoboda, James A., and Malcolm J. Thompson. Comparative effects of fatty acids on adult development in *Manduca sexta*. In Kabara 1989, chapter 4.

Ikawa, Miyoshi. Toxic and ecological effects of fatty acids on animals and microorganisms. In Kabara 1989, chapter 5.

Leung, Kam H. Modulation of cellular immunity by arachidonic acid metabolites. In Kabara 1989, chapter 6.

Kitagawa, Shuji. Regulatory functions of fatty acids on blood platelets. In Kabara 1989, chapter 7.

Pasternak, C. A., G. M. Alder, C. L. Bashford, and G. Menestrina. The role of lipids in permeability changes induced by toxins and other cytolytic agents. In Kabara 1989, chapter 8.

Fisher, Paul B., David Schachter, R. Allan Mufson, and Eliezer Huberman. The role of membrane lipid dynamics and translocation of protein kinase C in the induction of differentiation in human promyelocytic leukemic cells. In Kabara 1989, chapter 9.

Daniel, Larry W. Protein kinase C inhibition by alkyl-linked lipids. In Kabara 1989, chapter 10.

Houdebine, Louis-Marie, Michele Olliuier-Bousquet, Eue Deuinoy, and Paule Martel. Effect of phorbol esters and phospholipid derivatives on multiplication and differentiation of mammary cells. In Kabara 1989, chapter 11.

Trosko, James E., and Chia-Cheng Chang. Chemical tumor promoters, oncogenes and growth factors: Modulators of gap junctional intercellular communication. In Kabara 1989, chapter 12.

Aylsworth, Charles F. Inhibition of gap junction-mediated intercellular communication by unsaturated lipids: Potential involvement of protein kinase. In Kabara 1989, chapter 13.

Carroll, Kenneth K., E. Ann Jacobson, and Kathi A. James. Role of dietary fat in carcinogenesis. In Kabara 1989, chapter 14.

Welsch, Clifford W., Dietary fat and mammary gland development in the mature female BALB/c mouse. In Kabara 1989, chapter 15.

Reddy, Bandaru S. Dietary fat and colon cancer: Effect of type and amount of fat. In Kabara 1989, chapter 16.

Birt, Diane F. Effects of dietary fat on pancreatic carcinogenesis in the Syrian hamster. In Kabara 1989, chapter 17.

Yanagi, Susumu, Mariko Yamashita, Mitsuaki Sakamoto, Kyoko Kumazawa, and Shunsuke Imai. Comparative effects of butter, margarine, safflower oil and dextrin on mammary tumorigenesis in mice and rats. In Kabara 1989, chapter 18.

Cohen, L. A. Medium-chain triglycerides lack tumor-promoting effects in then-methylnitrosourea-induced mammary tumor model. In Kabara 1989, chapter 19.

Begin, Michel E. Selective antineoplastic effects of polyunsaturated fatty acids. In Kabara 1989, chapter 20.

Chapkin, Robert S., Scott D. Somers, and Kent L. Erickson. Effects of dietary fish oil on in vitro murine peritoneal macrophage cytolytic function. In Kabara 1989, chapter 21.

Garattini, Silvio, Roberto Fanelli, Alessandro Noseda, and Chiara Chiabrando. Prostaglandins and tumor growth and dissemination. In Kabara 1989, chapter 22.

Fukushima, Masanori. Prostaglandins A and J—Antitumor, antiviral activities and the mode of action. In Kabara 1989, chapter 23.

Ramachandran, C. K., and G. Melnykovych. Synthesis of mevalonate products in cells in culture effects of glucocorticoid steroids. In Kabara 1989, chapter 24.

Doyle, James W., Bruce D. Kabakoff, and Andrew A. Kandutsch. Isoprenoids and the cell cycle. In Kabara 1989, chapter 25.

Deliconstantinos, George, Gregory Skalkeas, and Gerhard R. F. Krueger. Effect of cholesterol binding on enzyme activity and fluidity of biomembranes: Studies of the consequences of cholesterol interaction with normal and leukemia cells. In Kabara 1989, chapter 26.

Holmes, Ross P. Effects of oxygenated sterols on cellular properties. In Kabara 1989, chapter 27.

Luu, Bang. Antitumoral and immunomodulating effects of oxygenated sterols: Interaction of oxygenated sterols with cell membranes. In Kabara 1989, chapter 28.

Zhang, H., K. H. Jones, W. B. Davis, R. L. Whisler, R. V. Panganamala, and D. G. Cornwell. Heterogeneity in lipid peroxides: Cellular arachidonic acid metabolism and DNA synthesis. In Kabara 1989, chapter 29.

O'Brien, Peter J., Hari Kaul, Larry McGirr, Diane Drolet, and Jose M. Silua. Molecular mechanisms for the involvement of the aldehydic metabolites of lipid peroxides in cytotoxicity and carcinogenesis. In Kabara 1989, chapter 30.

C) Selected References
from the Internet—Entrez Medline

Aebi, H. 1964. Vitamin D metabolism in caries. [In German.] *Bibl Nutr Dieta* 16:82–99.

American Urological Association Practice Guidelines Committee. 2003. AUA Guideline on the management of benign prostatic hyperplasia (BPH). *J Urol* 170 (2 Pt.1):530–547.

Andrews, C. H., and D. M. Hortsmann. 1949. Susceptibility of viruses to diethyl ether. *J Gen Microbial* 3:290.

Ascherio, A. 2002. Epidemiologic studies on dietary fats and coronary heart disease. *Am J Med* 113 (suppl):9S–12S.

Babayan, V. K. 1989. Sense and nonsense about fat in the diet. *Food Tech* (January):90.

Bach, A. C., and V. K. Babayan. 1982. Medium-chain triglycerides. *Am J Clin Nutr* 26:950.

Barry, M. A., D. E. Craven, T. A. Goularte, and D. A. Lichtenberg. 1984 (Sept). *Serratia marcescens* contamination of antiseptic soap containing triclosan: implications for nosocomial infection. *Infect Control* 5(9):427–430.

Basch, E., S. Gabard, and C. Ulbricht. 2003. Bitter melon *(Momordica charantia):* A review of efficacy and safety. *Am J Health Syst Pharm* 60:356–359.

Beuchat, L. R. 1980. Comparison of anti-Vibrio activities of potassium sorbate, sodium benzoate, and glycerol and sucrose esters of fatty acids. *Appl Environ Microbiol* 39 (6):1178–1182.

Bitman, J., D. L. Wood, M. Hamosh, and N. R. Mehta. 1983. Comparison of the lipid composition of breast milk from mothers of term and preterm infants. *Am J Clin Nutr* 38:300.

Blackburn, G. L. et al. 1989. A reevaluation of coconut oil's effect on serum cholesterol and atherogenesis. *J Philp Med Assoc* 202:1119.

Blough, H. A., and J. M. Tiffany. 1973. Lipids in viruses. *Adv Lipid Res* 11:267–339.

Boekholdt, S. M., C. E. Hack, M. S. Sandhu, R. Luben, S. A. Bingham, N. J. Wareham, R. J. Peters, J. W. Jukema, N. E. Day, J. J. Kastelein, and K. T. Shaw. 2006 (Aug). C-reactive protein levels and coronary artery disease incidence and mortality in apparently healthy men and women: the EPIC-Norfolk prospective population study 1993–2003. *Atherosclerosis* 187(2):415–422. E-pub Oct 28, 2005.

Boissoneault, G. A., and M. G. Hayek. 1992. Dietary fat, immunity, and inflammatory disease. In *Fatty Acids and Their Health Implications,* ed. Ching Kuang Chow. New York: Marcel Dekker.

Boyle, E., and J. B. German. 1996. Monoglycerides in membrane systems. *Crit Rev Food Sci Nutr* 36:785–805.

Boyle, P. 1994. New insights into the epidemiology and natural history of benign prostatic hyperplasia. *Prog Clin Biol Res* 386:3–18.

Burton, A. F. 1991. Oncolytic effects of fatty acids in mice and rats. *Am J Clin Nutr* 53: (4 Suppl):1082S–1086S.

Carrol, K. K. 1983. The role of fat in carcinogenesis. In *Dietary Fats and Health*, ed. E. G. Perkins and W. J. Visek, 710–720. Champaign, IL: American Oil Chemists' Society.

Ching Kuang Chow, ed. *Fatty Acids and Their Health Implications.* New York: Marcel Dekker.

Clarke, N. M., and J. T. May. 2000. Effect of antimicrobial factors in human milk on rhinoviruses and milk-borne cytomegalovirus in vitro. *J Med Microbiol* 49 (8):719–723.

Crouch, A. A., W. K. Seow, L. M. Whitman, and Y. H. Thong. 1991 (Sept-Oct). Effect of human milk and infant milk formula on adherence of Giardia intestinalis. *Trans R Soc Trop Med Hyg* 85(5):617–619.

De Pablo, M. A., and Gerardo Álvarez De Cienfuegos. 2000. Modulatory effects of dietary lipids on immune system functions. *Immunology and Cell Biology* 78:31–39.

Doyle, V. C. 2007. Nutrition and colorectal cancer risk: A literature review. *Gastroenterol Nurs* 30 (3):178–182.

Eady, E. A. 1998. Bacterial resistance in acne. *Dermatology* 196:59–66.

Eichholzer, M., H. B. Stahelin, F. Gutzwiller, E. Ludin, and F. Bernasconi. 2000. Association of low plasma cholesterol with mortality for cancer at various sites in men: 17-y follow-up of the prospective Basel study. *Am J Clin Nutr* 71(2):569–574.

Emilio, R. 2003. Intestinal absorption of triglyceride and cholesterol. Dietary and pharmacological inhibition to reduce cardiovascular risk. *Atherosclerosis* 151:357–359.

Enig, M. 1996. Health and nutritional benefits of functional food for the 21st century. *Coconut Today* 13:70.

Fieldsteel, A. H. 1974 (April). Nonspecific antiviral substances in human milk active against arbovirus and murine leukemia virus. *Cancer Res* 34(4):712–715.

Fox, J. G., and A. Lee. 1989. Gastric campylobacter-like organisms: Their role in gastric diseases in laboratory animals. *Lab Animal Sci* 39:543–553.

Gerber, G. S., D. Kuznetsov, B. C. Johnson, and J. D. Burstein. 2001. Randomized, double-blind, placebo-controlled trial of saw palmetto in men with lower urinary tract symptoms. *Urology* 58:960–964.

German, J.B., and C.J. Dillard. 2004 (Sept). Saturated fats: what dietary intake? *Am J Clin Nutr.* 80(3):550–59.

Goldberg, R. J., and J. A. Katz. 2007. A meta-analysis of the analgesic effects of omega-3 polyunsaturated fatty acid supplementation for inflammatory joint pain. *Pain* 129 (1–2): 210–223.

Grundy, S. M. 1994. Lipids and cardiovascular disease. In *Nutrition and Disease Update—Heart Disease,* eds. D. Kritchevsky and Kenneth K. Carroll. Champaign, IL: American Oil Chemists' Society.

Guinea, R., and L. Carrasco. 1991. Effects of fatty acids on lipid synthesis and viral RNA replication in poliovirus-infected cells. *Virology* 185:473.

Hardardóttir, I., and J. C. Kinsella. 1992. Increasing the dietary (n-3) to (n-6) polyunsaturated fatty acid ratio increases tumor necrosis factor production by murine resident peritoneal macrophages without an effect on elicited peritoneal macrophages. *J Nutr* 122(10):1942–1951.

Hopkins, P. N., and R. R. Williams. 1981. Risk factors in cardiovascular disease. *Athersclerosis* 40:1.

Hornung, B., E. Amtmann, and Gerhard Sauer. 1992. Medium chain-length fatty acids stimulate triacylglycerol synthesis in tissue culture cells. *Biochem Pharm* 43(2):175.

Hornung, B., E. Amtmann, and Gerhard Sauer. 1994. Lauric acid inhibits the maturation of vesicular stomatitis virus. *Virology* 75:353–361.

Howard, B. V., L. Van Horn, J. Hsia *et al.* 2006. Low-fat dietary pattern and risk of cardiovascular disease: The Women's Health Initiative Randomized Controlled Dietary Modification Trial. *JAMA* 295:655–666.

Isaacs, C. E., R. E. Litov, and H. Thormar. 1995. Antimicrobial activity of lipids added to human milk, infant formula, and bovine milk. *J Nutr Biochem* 6:362–366.

Isaacs, C. E., L. Rohan, W. Xu, J. H. Jia, T. Mietzner, and S. Hillier. 2006 (March). Inactivation of Herpes simplex virus clinical isolates by using a combination microbiocide. *Antimicrob Agents Chemother* 50(3):1063–1066.

Kaunitz, H. 1961. Reevaluation of some factors in arteriosclerosis. *Nature* 192:9.

Kaunitz, H. 1970. Nutritional properties of coconut oil. *J Am Oil Chem Soc* 47:462.

Kaunitz, H. 1983. Biological and therapeutic effects of MCT from coconut oil. *Coconut Today* 1(2): 27.

Kaunitz, H. 1988. Adaptive changes in arteriosclerosis, role of cholesterol. *Mech Ag Devel* 44:35–43.

Kaunitz, H. 1991. Is arteriosclerosis a life-prolonging adaptive factor? *Mechan Ag Devel* 57:137–144.

Kaunitz, H. 1995. Virally induced arteriosclerosis: Increased life expectancy? *Med Hypotheses* 45(4):335.

Kaunitz, H., C. A. Slaven, R. E. Johnson, and V. K. Babayan. 1959. Interrelations of linoleic acid with medium-chain and long-chain saturated triglycerides. *J Am Oil Chem Soc* 36:322–325.

Kaunitz, H., and C. S. Dayrit. 1992. Coconut oil consumption and coronary heart disease. *Philippine Journal of Coconut Studies* 17(2):18.

Kitahara, T., N. Koyam, J. Matsuda, Y. Aoyama, Y. Hirakata, S. Kamihara, S. Kohno, M. Nakashima, and H. Sasaki. 2004. Antimicrobial activity of saturated fatty acids and fatty amines against Methicillin-resistant *Staphylococcus aureus*. *Biol Pharm Bull* 27(9):1321–1326.

Kelley, D. S. 1996. Dietary fat and the immune response. *INFORM* 7(8):852–858.

Kohn, A., J. Gitelman, and M. Inbar. 1980. Interaction of polyunsaturated fatty acids with animal cells and enveloped viruses. *Antimicrob Agents Chemother* 189:962.

Konishi, T., H. Satsu, Y. Hatsugai, K. Aizawa, T. Inakuma, S. Nagata, S. Sakuda, H. Nagasawa, and M. Shimizu. 2004. Inhibitory effect of a bitter melon extract on the P-glycoprotein activity in intestinal Caco-2 cells. *British Journal of Pharmacology* 143:379–387.

Krizner, Ken. 2005. Complementary and alternative medicine is a $30 billion industry that has become more mainstream. *Managed Healthcare Executive* (February).

Lands, W. E. M., ed. 1987. *Polyunsaturated Fatty Acids and Eicosanoids.* Champaign, IL: American Oil Chemists' Society.

Li, Y., and H. E. Schellhorn. 2006. Can aging-related degenerative diseases be ameliorated through administration of vitamin C at pharmacological levels? *Med Hypotheses* (November).

Lyte, M., and M. Shinitzky. 1985. A special mixture for membrane fluidization. *Biochimica et biophysica acta* 821:133–138.

Marshall, B. J., J. A. Armstrong, D. B. McGeechie, and R. J. Glancy. 1985. Attempts to fulfill Koch's postulates for pyloric campylobacter. *Med J Aust* 142:436–439.

Marshall, B. J., and J. R. Warren. 1984. Unidentified curved bacilli on gastric epithelium in active chronic gastritis. *Lancet* 1:1311–1315.

McDonald, R., V. Dalle-Ore, and R. I. McDonald. 1984. Inhibition of sendai virus-induced hemolysis by long-chain fatty acids. *Virology* 134:103.

Meier, R. C. 2000. Antibiotics in the prevention and treatment of coronary heart disease. *Journal of Infectious Diseases* 181:S558–S562.

Melnick, J. L., B. L. Petrie, G. R. Dreesman, J. M. Burek, C. H. McCollum, and M. E. DeBakey. 1983. Cytomegalovirus antigen within human arterial smooth muscle cells. *Lancet* 2:644–647.

Melnick, J. L., *et al.* 1990. Possible role of cytomegalovirus in atherogenesis. *JAMA* 263:2204–2207.

Melnick, J. L., E. Adams, and M. E. DeBakey. 1993. Vol. 2, chapter 4 of *Frontiers of Virology,* eds. Y. Becker, G. Daral, and E. S. Huang. New York: Springer-Verlag.

Mendi, G. S., R. W. Wissler, R. T. Brindanstein, and F. T. Podhealaki. 1986. The effects of replacing coconut oil with corn oil on human serum lipid profiles and platelet-derived factors active in atherogenesis. *Nutrition Reports International* 40 (4 October).

Michihiro, S. 1987. One counterargument to the theory that tropical oils are harmful [In Japanese.] *Lipids* 40:48–51.

Morris, A., and G. Nicholson. 1987. Ingestion of *Campylobacter pyloris* causes gastritis and raised fasting gastric pH. *Am J Gastroenterol* 82:192–199.

Muhlestein, J. B. 1998. Chronic infection and coronary artery disease. *Science & Medicine* (November/December):16–25.

Muhlestein, J. B. 2002. Secondary prevention of coronary artery disease with antimicrobials: current status and future directions. *Am J Cardiovasc Drugs* 2(2):107–118.

Muldoon, M. F., and S. B. Manuck. 1990. Lowering cholesterol but not mortality. *BMJ* 11:301–309.

Muldoon, M. F., A. Marsland, J. D. Flory, B. S. Rabin, T. L. Whiteside, and S. B. Manuck. 1997. Immune system differences in men with hypo- or hypercholesterolemia. *Clin Immunol Immunopath* 84(2):145–149.

Muranushi, N., N. Takagi, S. Muranishi, and H. Sezaki. 1981. Effect of fatty acids and monoglycerides on permeability of lipid bilayer. *Chem Phys Lipids* 28(3):269–279.

Nickerson, K. W., V. C. Kramer, and J. J. Kabara. 1982. The effectiveness of Lauricidin preservative systems against detergent resistant Enterobactercloacae. *Soap Cosmet Specialities* (Feb 1982):50–58.

Nikoskelainen, Y., Y. L. Kalliomaki, K. Lapinleimu, M. Stenvik, and P. E. Halonen. 1983. Coxsackie B virus antibodies in myocardial infarction. *Acta Med Scand* 214:29–32.

Nizel, A. E. 1969. Dental caries: Protein, fats and carbohydrates. *N. Y. State Dent J* 35(2):71–81.

Parsonnett, J., G. D. Friedman, M. A. Vandersteen, Y. Chang, J. H. Vogelman, N. Orentreich, and R. K. Sibley. 1991. *Helicobacter pylori* infection and the risk of gastric carcinoma. *N Engl J Med* 325:1127–1131.

Perkins, E. G., and W. J. Visek, eds. 1983. *Dietary Fats and Health.* Champaign, IL: American Oil Chemists' Society.

Pestka, J. J., and M. F. Witt. 1985. An overview of immune function. *Food Tech* (February):83–90.

Petschow, B. W., R. P. Rosbatema, and L. L. Ford. 1996. Susceptibility of *Helicobacter pylori* to bactericidal properties of medium-chain mono-glycerides and free fatty acids. *Antimicro Agents and Chemother* 40:302–306.

Petschow, B. W., et al. 1998. Impact of medium-chain monoglycerides on intestinal colonization by *Vibrio cholerae* or enterotoxigenic *Escherichia coli*. *J Med Microbiol* 47(5):383–389.

Phillippoussis, F., C. Arguin, C. V. Mateo, A. M. Steff, and P. Hugo. 2003. Monoglycerides induce apoptosis in human leukemic cells while spar-ing normal peripheral blood mononuclear cells. *Blood* 101(1):292–294.

Preuss, H. G., B. Echard, A. Dadgar, N. Talpur, V. Manohar, M. Enig, D. Bagchi, and C. Ingram. 2005. Effects of essential oils and monolau-rin on *Staphylococcus aureus* in vitro and in vivo studies. *Toxicology Mech-anisms and Methods* 15:279–285.

Preuss, H. G., B. Echard, M. Enig, I. Brook, and T. B. Elliott. 2005 (April). Minimum inhibitory concentrations of herbal essential oils and mono-laurin for gram-positive and gram-negative bacteria. *Mol Cell Biochem* 272(1–2):29–34.

Prior, I. A., F. Davidson, E. C. Salmono, and Z. Czochanskaz. 1981. Cho-lesterol, coconuts and diets on Polynesian atolls: A natural experi-ment. *Am J Clin Nutr* 84:1552.

Projan, S. J., S. Brown-Skrobot, P. M. Schlievert, F. Vandenesch, and R. P. Novick. 1994. Glycerol monolaurate inhibits the production of beta-lactamase, toxic shock toxin-1, and other staphylococcal exoproteins by interfering with signal transduction. *J Bacteriol* 176:4204–4209.

Ravnskov, U. 1998. The questionable role of saturated and polyunsatu-rated fatty acids in cardiovascular disease. *J Clin Epidemiol* 51:443–460.

Ravnskov, U. 2002. Hypothesis out-of-date. The diet-heart idea. *J Clin Epidemiol* 55:1057–1063.

Reddy, B. S., and Y. Maeura. 1984. Tumor promotion of dietary fat in Azoxymethane-induced colon carcinogenesis in female F-344 rats. *Journal of the National Cancer Institute* 72:745–750.

Reiner, D. S., C. S. Wang, and F. D. Gillin. 1986 (Nov). Human milk kills *Giardia lamblia* by generating toxic lipolytic products. *J Infect Dis* 154(5):825–832.

Ridker, P. M., C. H. Hennekens, J. E. Buring, and N. Rifai. 2000. C-reactive protein and other markers of inflammation in the prediction of cardiovascular disease in women. *N Engl J Med* 342:836–843.

Ridker, P. M. 2005. C-reactive protein. *J Am Coll Cardiol* 46(1): 2–5.

Rosebury, T., and M. Karshan. 1939. Susceptibility to dental caries in the rat VIII. Further studies of the influence of vitamin D and of fats and fatty oils. *J Dent Res* 18:189–202.

Ross, R. 1993. The pathogenesis of atherosclerosis: A perspective for the 1990s. *Nature* 362:801.

Ruzin, A., and R. P. Novick. 1998. Glycerol monolaurate inhibits induction of vancomycin resistance in *Enterococcus faecalis. J Bacteriol* 180:182–185.

Sadikot, S. M. 1994. Beneficial effects of coconut oil. *Ind Coco J* 25(1):2–13.

Schlievert, P. M., J. R. Deringer, M. H. Kims, S. J. Projan, and R. P. Novick. 1992. Effect of glycerol monolaurate on bacterial growth and toxin production. *Antimicrob Agents Chemother* 36:626–631.

Sheu, C. W., and E. Freese. 1972. Effects of fatty acids on growth and envelope proteins of *Bacillus subtilis. J Bacteriol* 111 (2):516–524.

Shimada, H., V. E. Tyler, and J. L. McLaughlin. 1997. Biologically active acylglycerides from the berries of saw-palmetto *(Serenoa repens). J Nat Prod* 60(4):417–418.

Smith, R. L. 1989. Dietary lipids and heart disease. *American Clinical Laboratory* (November):26.

Stehbens, W. E. 1989. The controversial role of dietary cholesterol and hypercholesterolemia. *Pathology* 21:213–221.

Stehbens, W. E. 1989. *The Lipid Hypothesis of Atherogenesis.* Austin, TX: R. G. Landes.

Sterling, V., and B. S. Mead. 1937. A study of the bactericidal, bacteriostatic and peptizing action of certain dentifrices. *J Dent Res* 16(1):41–50.

Stock, C. C., and T. Francis, Jr. 1940. The inactivation of the virus of epidemic influenza by soaps. *J Exp Med* 77:661.

Stock, C. C., and T. Francis, Jr. 1943. Additional studies of the inactivation of the virus of epidemic influenza by soaps. *J Immunol* 47:303.

Stock, C. C. and T. Francis, Jr. 1943. The inactivation of the virus of lymphocytic choriomeningitis by soaps. *J Exp Med* 77:323.

Schuster, G. S., T. R. Dirksen, A. E. Ciarlone, G. Burnett, M. T. Reynolds, and M. T. Lankford. 1980. Anticaries and antiplaque potential of free-fatty acids in vitro and in vivo. *Pharmacol Ther Dent* 5(1-2):25–33.

Suarez, E. C. 1999. Relations of trait depression and anxiety to low lipid and lipoprotein concentrations in healthy young adult women. *Psychosom Med* 61(3):273–279.

Suller, M. T. E., and A. D. Russell. 2000. Triclosan and antibiotic resistance in *Staphyloccus aureus*. *Journal of Antimicrobial Chemotherapy* 46:11–18.

Tannenbaum, A. 1942. The genesis and growth of tumors: III. Effects of high-fat diets. *Cancer Res* 2:468–475.

Thampan, P. K. 1994. *Facts and Fallacies about Coconut Oil*. Jakarta: Asian and Pacific Coconut Community.

Thomas, Paul, and J. K. Mukkaden. 1995. Is coconut oil consumption a major risk factor for coronary artery disease? *Ind Coco J* 32(7):41.

Thormar, H., C. E. Isaacs, H. Brown, M. R. Barshutzky, and T. Pessolano. 1987. Inactivation of enveloped viruses and killing of cells by fatty acids and monoglycerides. *Antimicrob Agents Chemother* 31:27–31.

Thormar, H., G. Bergsson, E. Gunnarsson, G. Georgsson, M. Witvrouw, O. Steingrimsson, E. De Clercq, and T. Kristmundsdottir. 1999. Hydrogels containing monocaprin have potent microbiocidal activities against sexually transmitted viruses and bacteria in vitro. *Sex Transm Infect* 75:181–185.

Timms, R. 1999. Fat or fiction: Saturated fat defended. *Inform* 10(9).

Tomlinson, S. S., and K. K. Mangione. 2005. Potential adverse effects of statins on muscle. *Phys Ther* 85(5):459–465.

Tomoko, Konishi, et al. 2004. Inhibitory effect of a bitter melon extract on the P-glycoprotein activity in intestinal Caco-2 cells. *British Journal of Pharmacology* 143:379–387.

Tsuchido, T., Y. H. Ahn, M. Takano. 1987. Lysis of *Bacillus subtilis* cells by glycerol and sucrose esters of fatty acids. *Appl Environ Microbiol* 53(3):505–508.

Upledger, J. E. 2000. *Craniosacral Therapy and the Immune Response*. Berkeley, CA: North Atlantic Books.

Upledger, J. E. 2003. *Cell Talk*. Berkeley, CA: North Atlantic Books.

Vadhat, K., S. M. Jafari, R. Pazoki, and I. Nabipour. 2007. Concurrent increased high sensitivity C-reactive protein and chronic infections are associated with coronary artery disease: A population-based study. *Indian J Med Sci* 61(3):135–143.

Vanderbelt, J. 1945. Nutritive value of coconut. *Nature* 156:174–175.

Ved, H. S., E. Gustow, and R. A. Pieringer. 1984 (Aug). Inhibition of peptidoglycan synthesis of *Streptococcus faecium* ATCC 9790 and *Streptococcus mutans* BHT by the antibacterial agent dodecylglycerol. *Biosci Rep* 4(8):659–664.

Ved, H. S., E. Gustow, and R. A. Pieringer. 1990 (Feb). Synergism between penicillin G and the antimicrobial ether lipid, rac-1-dodecylglycerol, acting below its critical micelle concentration. *Lipids* 25(2):119–121.

Verghese, E. J. 1952. Food value of coconut products. *Ind Coco J* 5:119.

Visser, M. R., and C. M. Vercellotti. 1993. Herpes simplex virus and atherosclerosis. *Eur Heart J* 14 (Suppl K):39–42.

Vojdani, Aristo. The role of periodontal disease and other infections in the pathogenesis of atherosclerosis and systemic diseases. *Immunosciences Lab,* no. 209:52–56.

Wanke, C. A., D. Pleskow, P. C. Degirolami, B. B. Lambl, K. Merkel, S. Akrabawi. 1996. A medium-chain triglyceride-based diet in patients with HIV and chronic diarrhea reduces diarrhea and malabsorption: A prospective, controlled trial. *Nutrition* 12 (11–12):766–771.

Wanten, G. J., and P. C. Calder. 2007. Immune modulation by parenteral lipid emulsions. *Am J Clin Nutr* 85(5):1171–1184.

Welsh, J. K., and J. T. May. 1979. Anti-infective properties of breast milk. *J Pediatr* 94:1–9.

Welsh, J. K., and J. T. May. 1981. Effect on Semliki Forest virus and Coxsackie virus B4 on lipids common to human milk. *J Food Safety* 99–107.

Williams, K. A., B. R. Schemehorn, J. L. McDonald, Jr., G. K. Stookey, and S. Katz. 1982. Influence of selected fatty acids upon plaque formation and caries in the rat. *Arch Oral Biol* 27(12):1027–1031.

Glossary of Biochemical and Medical Terms

Acetylation—the addition of an acetyl group (-COCH3) to a molecule.

Acidic—having a pH of less than 7.

Acute—having a short and relatively severe course.

AIDS—Acquired Immune Deficiency Syndrome. AIDS is believed to be caused by the Human Immunodeficiency Virus (HIV), which attacks the immune system, leaving the infected individual vulnerable to opportunistic infection.

Alkaline—basic; having a pH of more than 7.

Alkaloid—a plant-derived compound that is biologically active, contains a nitrogen in a heterocyclic ring, is alkaline, has a complex structure, and is of limited distribution in the plant kingdom.

Amino acids—organic (carbon-containing) molecules that serve as the building blocks of proteins.

Anaphylaxis—a rapidly developing and severe systemic allergic reaction.

Anemia—the condition of having less than the normal number of red blood cells or hemoglobin in the blood.

Anion—a negatively charged ion.

Angiogenesis—the formation of new blood vessels.

Antagonist—a substance that counteracts or nullifies the biological effects of another, such as a compound that binds to a receptor but does not elicit a biological response.

Antibodies—specialized proteins produced by white blood cells (lymphocytes) that recognize and bind to foreign proteins or pathogens in order to neutralize them or mark them for destruction.

Anticonvulsant—a class of medication used to prevent seizures.

Antigen—a substance that is capable of eliciting an immune response.

Antioxidant—any substance that prevents or reduces damage caused by reactive oxygen species (ROS) or reactive nitrogen species (RNS).

Apoptosis—one of the main types of programmed cell death (PCD). As such, it is a process of deliberate life relinquishment by an unwanted cell in a multicellular organism.

Atherosclerosis—an inflammatory disease resulting in the accumulation of cholesterol-laden plaque in artery walls. Rupture of atherosclerotic plaque results in clot formation, which may result in myocardial infarction or ischemic stroke.

Autoimmune disease—a condition in which the body's immune system reacts against its own tissues.

Bacteria—single-celled organisms that can exist independently, symbiotically (in cooperation with another organism), or parasitically (dependent upon another organism, sometimes to the detriment of the host organism). Examples of bacteria include acidophilus (found in yogurt), streptococcus (the cause of strep throat), and *E. coli* (a normal intestinal bacteria, as well as a disease-causing agent).

Benign prostatic hyperplasia (BPH)—the term used to describe a noncancerous enlargement of the prostate.

Bioavailability—the fraction of an administered (or consumed) compound that reaches the systemic circulation and is transported to the site of action (target tissue).

Biomarker—a physical, functional, or biochemical indicator of a physiological or disease process.

Bipolar disorder—characterized by severe alterations in mood. During "manic" episodes, a person may experience extreme elevation in energy level and mood (euphoria) or extreme agitation and irritability. Episodes of depressed mood are also common in bipolar disorder.

Bronchitis, chronic—standing inflammation of the airways, characterized by excess production of sputum, leading to a chronic cough and obstruction of air flow. Cigarette smoking is the most common cause of chronic bronchitis.

Cancer—refers to abnormal cells, which have a tendency to grow uncontrollably and to metastasize or spread to other areas of the body. Cancer can involve any tissue of the body and can have different forms in one tissue. Cancer is a group of more than a hundred different diseases.

Carbohydrate—chemically, carbohydrates are neutral compounds composed of carbon, hydrogen, and oxygen. Carbohydrates come in simple forms known as sugars and complex forms such as starches and fiber.

Carboxylation—the introduction of a carboxyl group (-COOH) or carbon dioxide into a compound.

Carcinogenesis—the formation of cancer cells from normal cells.

Case reports—individual observations based on small numbers of subjects. This type of research cannot indicate causality but may indicate areas for further research.

Catalyze—to increase the speed of a chemical reaction without changing the overall reaction process. See *Enzyme*.

Cation—a positively charged ion.

Cell adhesion molecules—molecules on the outside surfaces of cells that bind to other cells or to the extracellular matrix (material surrounding cells). Cell adhesion molecules influence many important functions, including the entry of immune cells into the arterial wall.

Cell signaling—communication among individual cells so as to coordinate their behavior to benefit the organism as a whole. Cell-signaling systems elucidated in animal cells include cell-surface and intracellular receptor proteins.

Chelate—to combine a metal with an organic molecule to form a ring-like structure known as a chelate. Chelation of a metal may inhibit or enhance its bioavailability.

Chemotherapy—literally, treatment with drugs or chemicals. Commonly used to describe the systemic use of drugs to kill cancer cells (a form of cancer treatment).

Cholesterol—a compound that is an integral structural component of cell membranes and a precursor in the synthesis of steroid hormones.

Chromosome—a structure in the nucleus of a cell that contains genes. Chromosomes are composed of DNA and associated proteins.

Chylomicrons—triglyceride-rich lipoproteins that deliver dietary triglycerides from the intestine to the tissues immediately after a meal.

Chylomicronemia—above-normal quantity of microscopic particles containing fats, cholesterol, phospholipids, and protein, formed in the small intestine and absorbed into the blood during digestion.

Clinical trial—an intervention trial generally used to evaluate the efficacy and/or safety of a treatment or intervention in human participants.

Colon—the portion of the large intestine that extends from the end of the small intestine to the rectum.

Congestive heart failure (CHF)—a condition in which the heart loses the ability to pump blood efficiently enough to meet the demands of the body.

Coronary heart disease (CHD)—also known as coronary artery disease and coronary disease, coronary heart disease is the result of atherosclerosis of the coronary arteries.

Corticosteroid—any of the steroid hormones made by the cortex (outer layer) of the adrenal gland. Cortisol is a corticosteroid.

C-reactive protein (CRP)—a protein that is produced in the liver in response to inflammation. CRP is a biomarker of inflammation that is strongly associated with the risk of cardiovascular events, such as myocardial infarction and stroke.

Crohn's disease—an inflammatory bowel disease that usually affects the lower part of the small intestine or upper part of the colon, but may affect any part of the gastrointestinal tract.

Cytoplasm—the contents of a cell, excluding the nucleus.

De novo synthesis—the formation of an essential molecule from simple precursor molecules.

Dental caries—cavities or holes in the outer two layers of a tooth—the enamel and the dentin. Dental caries are caused by bacteria that metabolize carbohydrates (sugars) to form organic acids that dissolve tooth enamel.

Dermatitis—inflammation of the skin. This term is often used to describe a skin rash.

Diabetes mellitus—a chronic metabolic disease characterized by abnormally high blood glucose (sugar) levels, resulting from the inability of the body to produce or respond to insulin. Type 1 diabetes mellitus, formerly known as insulin-dependent or juvenile-onset diabetes, is usually the result of autoimmune destruction of the insulin-secreting beta cells of the pancreas. The most common form of diabetes is type 2 diabetes mellitus, formerly known as noninsulin-dependent or adult-onset diabetes, which develops when the tissues of the body become less sensitive to insulin secreted by the pancreas.

Diverticulitis—inflammation or infection of diverticula in the colon. Characterized by abdominal pain, fever, and constipation.

DNA (deoxyribonucleic acid)—a double-stranded nucleic acid composed of many nucleotides. The nucleotides in DNA are each composed of a nitrogen-containing base (adenine, guanine, cytosine, or thymine), a 5-carbon sugar (deoxyribose), and a phosphate group. The sequence of bases in DNA encodes the genetic information required to synthesize proteins.

Double blind—refers to a study in which neither the investigators administering the treatment nor the participants know which participants are receiving the experimental treatment and which are receiving the placebo.

Eicosanoids—chemical messengers derived from 20-carbon polyunsaturated fatty acids, such as arachidonic acid and eicosapentaenoic acid. Eicosanoids play critical roles in immune and inflammatory responses.

Electron—a stable atomic particle with a negative charge.

Emulsifier—a substance that allows oil and water to be combined into a stable system without separation.

Enamel—the hard, white, outermost layer of a tooth.

Endocrine system—the glands and parts of glands that secrete hormones which integrate and control the body's metabolic activity. Endocrine glands include the pituitary, thyroid, parathyroids, adrenals, pancreas, ovaries, and testes.

Endogenous—arising from within the body. Endogenous synthesis refers to the synthesis of a compound by the body.

Enterocytes—cells that line the luminal (inner) surface of the intestine.

Enzyme—a biological catalyst. That is, a substance that increases the speed of a chemical reaction without being changed in the overall process. Enzymes are vitally important to the regulation of the chemistry of cells and organisms.

Epilepsy—also known as seizure disorder. Individuals with epilepsy experience seizures, which are the result of uncontrolled electrical activity in the brain. A seizure may cause a physical convulsion, minor physical signs, thought disturbances, or a combination of symptoms.

Ester—the product of a reaction between a carboxylic acid and an alcohol that involves the elimination of water. For example, the ester monolaurin is the product of a reaction between lauric acid and glycerol.

Etiology—the causes or origin of a disease.

Fatty acid—an organic acid molecule consisting of a chain of carbon molecules and a carboxylic acid (COOH) group.

Free radical—a very reactive atom or molecule typically possessing a single unpaired electron.

Gastrointestinal—referring to or affecting the digestive tract, which includes the mouth, pharynx (throat), esophagus, stomach, and intestines.

Gene—a region of DNA that controls a specific hereditary characteristic, usually corresponding to a single protein.

Gene expression—the process by which the information coded in genes (DNA) is converted to proteins and other cellular structures. Expressed genes include those that are transcribed to mRNA and translated to protein, as well as those that are only transcribed to RNA (e.g. ribosomal and transfer RNAs).

Gluconeogenesis—the production of glucose from non-carbohydrate precursors, such as amino acids (the building blocks of proteins).

Glycogen—a large polymer (repeating units) of glucose molecules, used to store energy in cells, especially muscle and liver cells.

Glycoside—a compound containing a sugar molecule that can be cleaved by hydrolysis to a sugar and a nonsugar component (aglycone).

HDL—high-density lipoprotein. HDLs transport cholesterol from the tissues to the liver, where it can be eliminated in bile. HDL cholesterol is considered good cholesterol, because higher blood levels of HDL cholesterol are associated with lower risk of heart disease.

Hepatitis—literally, inflammation of the liver. Hepatitis caused by a virus is known as viral hepatitis. Other causes of hepatitis include toxic chemicals and alcohol abuse.

HIV—Human Immunodeficiency Virus, the virus that causes AIDS.

Homocysteine—a sulfur-containing amino acid, which is an inter-
mediary in the metabolism of another sulfur-containing amino
acid, methionine. Elevated homocysteine levels in the blood
have been associated with increased risk of cardiovascular disease.

Human papilloma virus (HPV)—a group of viruses that may cause
papillomas (growths or warts) on the skin or other parts of the
body, including the genitals and the larynx (voice box). Infection with particular strains of HPV is associated with increased risk
of cervical cancer.

Hydrolysis—cleavage of a chemical bond by the addition of water.
In hydrolysis reactions, a large compound may be broken down
into smaller compounds when a molecule of water is added.

Hyperglyceridemia—above-normal triglyceride levels in the blood.

Hypothesis—an educated guess or proposition that is advanced as
a basis for further investigation. A hypothesis must be subjected
to an experimental test to determine its validity.

Idiopathic—of unknown cause.

Inflammation—a response to injury or infection, characterized by
redness, heat, swelling, and pain. Physiologically, the inflammatory response involves a complex series of events, leading to
the migration of white blood cells to the inflamed area.

In vitro—literally, "in glass," referring to a test or research done in
the test tube, outside a living organism.

In vivo—"inside a living organism." An *in vivo* assay evaluates a biological process occurring inside the body.

Ion—an atom or group of atoms that carries a positive or negative
electric charge as a result of having lost or gained one or more
electrons.

Ion channel—a protein embedded in a cell membrane that serves as a crossing point for the regulated transfer of an ion or a group of ions across the membrane.

Isomers—compounds that have the same numbers and kinds of atoms but differ in the way the atoms are arranged.

Ketone bodies—any of three acidic chemicals (acetate, acetoacetate, and beta-hydroxybutyrate). Ketone bodies may accumulate in the blood (ketosis) when the body has inadequate glucose to use for energy and must increase the use of fat for fuel. Ketone bodies are acidic, and very high levels in the blood are toxic and may result in ketoacidosis.

Lauric acid—12-chain fatty acid.

Lauricidin®—trade name for the monoglyceride monolaurin /glyceryl monolaurate.

LDL (low-density lipoprotein)—LDLs transport cholesterol from the liver to the tissues of the body. Elevated serum LDL cholesterol is associated with increased cardiovascular disease risk.

Leukemia—an acute or chronic form of cancer that involves the blood-forming organs. Leukemia is characterized by an abnormal increase in the number of white blood cells in the tissues of the body, with or without a corresponding increase of those in the circulating blood; the disease is classified according to the type of white blood cell most prominently involved.

Leukocytes—white blood cells. Leukocytes are part of the immune system. Monocytes, lymphocytes, neutrophils, basophils, and eosinophils are different types of leukocytes.

Leukotrienes—cell-signaling molecules involved in inflammation.

Lipid peroxidation—the process by which lipids are oxidatively modified; so named because lipid hydroperoxides are formed in the process.

Lipids—a chemical term for fats. Lipids found in the human body include fatty acids, phospholipids, triglycerides, and cholesterol.

Lipoproteins—particles composed of lipids and protein that allow for the transport of lipids through the bloodstream. A lipoprotein particle is composed of an outer layer of phospholipids, which renders it soluble in water, and a hydrophobic core that contains triglycerides and cholesterol esters. Types of lipoproteins are distinguished by their surface proteins (apoproteins), their size, and the types and amounts of lipids they contain.

Lipoxygenases—catalyze the formation of leukotrienes from eicosanoids, such as arachidonic acid and eicosapentaenoic acid (EPA).

Lymphocyte—a type of leukocyte (white blood cell) that plays important roles in the immune system. T lymphocytes (T cells) differentiate into cells that can kill infected cells or activate other cells in the immune system. B lymphocytes (B cells) differentiate into cells that produce antibodies.

Malignant—cancerous.

Meta-analysis—a statistical technique used to combine the results from different studies to obtain a quantitative estimate of the overall effect of a particular intervention or exposure on a defined outcome.

Metabolism—the sum of the processes (reactions) by which a substance is assimilated and incorporated into the body, or detoxified and excreted from the body.

Metabolite—a compound derived from the metabolism of another compound.

Metastasize—to spread from one part of the body to another. Cancer is said to metastasize when it spreads from the primary site of origin to a distant anatomical site.

Mitochondria—energy-producing structures within cells. Mitochondria possess two sets of membranes: a smooth continuous outer membrane, and an inner membrane arranged in folds. Among other critical functions, mitochondria convert nutrients into energy via the electron transport chain.

Monounsaturated fatty acid—a fatty acid with only one double bond between carbon atoms.

Mutation—a change in a gene; in other words, a change in the sequence of base pairs in the DNA that makes up a gene. Mutations in a gene may or may not result in an altered gene product.

Necrosis—unprogrammed cell death, in which cells break open and release their contents, promoting inflammation. Necrotic cell death may be the result of injury, infection, or infarction.

Neutrophils—white blood cells that internalize and destroy pathogens, such as bacteria. Neutrophils are also called polymorphonuclear leukocytes because they are white blood cells with multi-lobed nuclei.

Nucleic acids—DNA (deoxyribonucleic acid) and RNA (ribonucleic acid) are the two types; they are long polymers of nucleotides.

Nucleotides—subunits of nucleic acids. Nucleotides are composed of a nitrogen-containing base (adenine, guanine, cytosine, uracil, or thymine), a 5-carbon sugar (ribose or deoxyribose), and one or more phosphate groups.

Nucleus—a membrane-bound cellular organelle, containing DNA organized into chromosomes.

Optimum health—in addition to freedom from disease, the ability of an individual to function physically and mentally at his or her best.

Organelles—specialized components of cells, such as mitochondria or lysosomes, so named because they are analogous to organs of the body since organelles are also important parts of a whole (the cell).

Oxidative stress—a condition in which the effects of prooxidants (e.g. free radicals, reactive oxygen, and reactive nitrogen species) exceed the ability of antioxidant systems to neutralize them.

Peptic ulcer disease—characterized by ulcers or breakdown of the inner lining of the stomach or duodenum. Common risk factors for peptic ulcer disease include the use of nonsteroidal anti-inflammatory drugs (NSAIDs) and infection with *Helicobacter pylori.*

Peptide—a chain of amino acids. A protein is made up of one or more peptides.

Peptidoglycans—a large molecule (peptide bound to a carbohydrate) found in the walls of bacteria to provide their strength and shape.

pH—a measure of acidity or alkalinity.

Pharmacokinetics—the study of the absorption, distribution, metabolism, and elimination of drugs and other compounds.

Pharmacologic dose—the dose or intake level of a nutrient many times the level associated with the prevention of deficiency or the maintenance of health. A pharmacologic dose is generally associated with the treatment of a disease state and is usually at least ten times greater than that needed to prevent deficiency.

Phase I clinical trial—an experimental study in a small group of people aimed at determining bioavailability, optimal dose, safety, and early evidence of the efficacy of a new therapy.

Phase II clinical trial—tests how effective a new drug or procedure is against a particular medical problem.

Phase III trial—compares a promising new drug, new combination of drugs, or new procedure with the best standard treatment. Phase III trials typically involve large numbers of patients, usually hundreds or thousands. A patient in a Phase III trial is randomly assigned to receive either the new treatment or the best existing treatment.

Phase IV trial—asks new questions about standard treatments. A Phase IV trial might test how a newly approved drug works together with other effective drugs, or with surgery and/or radiation therapy.

Phospholipids—lipids in which phosphoric acid as well as fatty acids are attached to a glycerol backbone. Phospholipids are important structural components of cell membranes.

Physiologic dose—the dose or intake level of a nutrient associated with the prevention of deficiency or the maintenance of health. A physiologic dose of a nutrient is not generally greater than that which could be achieved through a conscientious diet, as opposed to the use of supplements.

Placebo—an inert treatment that is given to a control group while the experimental group is given the active treatment. Placebo-controlled studies are conducted to make sure that the results are due to the experimental treatment, rather than to another factor associated with participating in the study.

Pneumonia—a disease of the lungs characterized by inflammation and accumulation of fluid in the lungs. Pneumonia may be caused by infectious agents (e.g. viruses or bacteria) or by inhalation of certain irritants.

Polymer—a large molecule formed by combining many similar smaller molecules (monomers) in a regular pattern.

Precursor—a molecule that is an ingredient, reactant, or intermediate in a synthetic pathway for a particular product.

Prooxidant—an atom or molecule that promotes oxidation of another atom or molecule by accepting electrons. Examples of prooxidants include free radicals, reactive oxygen species (ROS), and reactive nitrogen species (RNS).

Prostaglandins—cell-signaling molecules involved in inflammation. Cyclooxygenases catalyze the formation of prostaglandins from eicosanoids such as arachidonic acid (AA, omega-6 polyunsaturated fatty acid) and eicosapentaenoic acid (EPA, omega-3 polyunsaturated fatty acid).

Prostate—a gland in men, located at the base of the bladder and surrounding the urethra. The prostate produces fluid that forms part of semen. If the prostate becomes enlarged it may exert pressure on the urethra and cause urinary symptoms. Prostate cancer is one of the most common types of cancer in men.

Prostate-specific antigen (PSA)—a compound normally secreted by the prostate that can be measured in the blood. If prostate cancer is developing, the prostate secretes larger amounts of PSA. Blood tests for PSA are used to screen for prostate cancer and to follow up on prostate cancer treatment.

Protein—a complex organic molecule composed of amino acids in a specific order. The order is determined by the sequence of nucleic acids in a gene coding for the protein. Proteins are required for the structure, function, and regulation of the body's cells, tissues, and organs; and each protein has unique functions.

Proton—an elementary particle identical to the nucleus of a hydrogen atom, that along with neutrons is a constituent of all other atomic nuclei. A proton carries a positive charge equal and opposite to that of an electron.

Psoriasis—A chronic skin condition often resulting in a red, scaly rash located over the surfaces of the elbows, knees, scalp, and around or in the ears, navel, genitals, or buttocks. Approximately 10–15% of patients with psoriasis develop joint inflammation (psoriatic arthritis). Psoriasis is thought to be an autoimmune condition.

Randomized controlled trial (RCT)—a clinical trial with at least one active treatment group and a control (placebo) group. In RCTs, participants are chosen for the experimental and control groups at random, and are not told whether they are receiving the active or placebo treatment until the end of the study. This type of study design can provide evidence of causality.

Randomized design—an experiment in which participants are chosen for the experimental and control groups at random, in order to reduce bias caused by self-selection into experimental and control groups. This type of study design can provide evidence of causality.

Receptor—a specialized molecule inside or on the surface of a cell that binds a specific chemical (ligand). Ligand binding usually results in a change in activity within the cell.

Redox reaction—another term for an oxidation-reduction reaction. A redox reaction is any reaction in which electrons are removed from one molecule or atom and transferred to another molecule or atom. In such a reaction one substance is oxidized (loses electrons) while the other is reduced (gains electrons).

Restenosis—with respect to the coronary arteries, restenosis refers to the reocclusion of a coronary artery after it has been dilated using coronary angioplasty.

RNA (ribonuceic acid)—a single-stranded nucleic acid composed of many nucleotides. The nucleotides in RNA are composed of a nitrogen-containing base (adenine, guanine, cytosine, or uracil), a 5-carbon sugar (ribose), and a phosphate group. RNA functions in the translation of the genetic information encoded in DNA to proteins.

Saturated fatty acid—a fatty acid with no double bonds between carbon atoms. There are three groups or types: short-, medium-, and long-chain saturated fatty acids.

Seizure—uncontrolled electrical activity in the brain, which may produce a physical convulsion, minor physical signs, thought disturbances, or a combination of symptoms.

Signal transduction pathway—a cascade of events that allows a signal outside a cell to result in a functional change inside the cell. Signal transduction pathways play important roles in regulating numerous cellular functions in response to changes in a cell's environment.

Steroid—a molecule related to cholesterol. Many important hormones, such as estrogen and testosterone, are steroids.

Substrate—a reactant in an enzyme-catalyzed reaction.

Supplement—a substance with particular nutritional value for better health.

Syndrome—a combination of symptoms that occur together and indicate a specific condition or disease.

Synergistic—when the effect of two treatments together is greater than the sum of the effects of the two individual treatments.

Systolic blood pressure—the highest arterial pressure measured during the heartbeat cycle, and the first number in a blood pressure reading (e.g. 120/80).

Threshold—the point at which a physiological effect begins to be produced: for example, the degree of stimulation of a nerve that produces a response, or the level of a chemical in the diet that results in a disease.

Topical—applied to the skin or other body surface.

Total Parenteral Nutrition (TPN)—intravenous (IV) feeding that provides patients with essential nutrients when they are too ill to eat normally.

Transcription (DNA transcription)—the process by which one strand of DNA is copied into a complementary sequence of RNA.

Translation (RNA translation)—the process by which the sequence of nucleotides in a messenger RNA molecule directs the incorporation of amino acids into a protein.

Triglycerides—lipids consisting of three fatty acid molecules bound to a glycerol backbone. Triglycerides are the principal form of fat in the diet, although they are also synthesized endogenously. Triglycerides are stored in adipose tissue and represent the principal storage form of fat. Elevated serum triglycerides are a risk factor for cardiovascular disease.

Tuberculosis—an infection caused by the bacteria *Mycobacteria tuberculosis.* Many people infected with tuberculosis have no symptoms because it is dormant. Once active, tuberculosis may cause damage to the lungs and other organs. Active tuberculosis is also contagious and is spread through inhalation. Treatment of tuberculosis involves taking antibiotics and vitamins for at least six months.

Typhoid—an infectious disease, spread by the contamination of food or water supplies with the bacteria called *Salmonella typhi.* Food and water can be contaminated directly by sewage or indirectly by flies or poor hygiene. Though rare in the U.S., it is common in some parts of the world. Symptoms include fever, abdominal pain, diarrhea, and a rash. It is treated with antibiotics and intravenous fluids. Vaccination is recommended to those traveling to areas where typhoid is common.

Unsaturated fatty acid—a fatty acid with at least one double bond between carbons.

Vesicle—literally a small bag or pouch. Inside a cell, a vesicle is a small organelle surrounded by its own membrane.

Virus—a microorganism that cannot grow or reproduce apart from a living cell. Viruses invade living cells and use the synthetic processes of infected cells to survive and replicate.

Vitamin—an organic (carbon-containing) compound necessary for normal physiological function that cannot be synthesized in adequate amounts and must therefore be obtained in the diet.

Index

About the Author

Dr. JON J. KABARA, BS, MS, PhD

Dr. Jon Kabara was a professor at the University of Detroit (ten years) and Michigan State University (MSU) for some twenty years and is now Professor Emeritus from MSU. Consultant to private industries, universities, and government agencies, he continues to write and give seminars on the pharmacological effects of lipids.

His professional career began in 1948 as a research assistant at the University of Illinois Department of Biochemistry. Six years after graduation from the University of Chicago, he received his full professorship at the University of Detroit (1965). In 1969, as Professor and Associate Dean, he helped establish a new private College of Osteopathic Medicine in Michigan, which became the first affiliated school of Osteopathic Medicine at a major university (Michigan State University).

His many achievements are listed in:

American Men of Science
Leaders in American Science
World's Who's Who in Science
Outstanding Educators of America
Two Thousand Men of Achievement
20th Century Award for Achievement
Who's Who in Medicine and Healthcare
International Man of the Year 1996–1997

Who's Who in Technology Today, 4th Edition
International Who's Who in Community Service
Who's Who in America (Fifty-Fourth Edition, 2000)

Dr. Kabara has been honored with sixteen scholarships or awards, has had many (thirty) research sponsors, and has been granted more than sixteen U.S. and foreign patents. He is credited with over two hundred publications including book chapters or books.